Talk Behavior to Me

Talk Behavior to Me provides a unique and comprehensive resource for those seeking to understand the science of behavior analysis. The publication features direct translations of the 150 most commonly used terms in the field, making it the first of its kind to provide clear and accessible explanations of behavior analytic jargon.

One of the book's standout features is its coverage of the many branches of behavior analysis, including applications in sports, fitness, forensics, organizational behavior management, public health, environmental sustainability, animal behavior training, and more. With this breadth of coverage, the book offers a valuable resource for practitioners and scholars alike, providing a single source for understanding the full range of behavior analytic practices. To further support readers, it includes illustrations throughout, which serve to clarify complex concepts and deepen the reader's understanding. Additionally, each chapter includes tips and lessons for the practical application of concepts.

Its accessible language, practical examples, and comprehensive coverage make *Talk Behavior to Me* an essential addition to the library of scholars, practitioners, and students alike.

Kendall Ryndak Samuel is a board-certified behavior analyst (BCBA) who has worked in various sub-specialties of behavior analysis, including dissemination, behavioral sports psychology, organizational behavior management, and autism.

Talk Behavior to Me

The Routledge Dictionary of the
Top 150 Behavior Analytic Terms
and Translations

Kendall Ryndak Samuel, BCBA

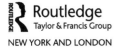

Routledge
Taylor & Francis Group

NEW YORK AND LONDON

Cover image: Getty Images © L-TOP

First published 2025
by Routledge
605 Third Avenue, New York, NY 10158

and by Routledge
4 Park Square, Milton Park, Abingdon, Oxon OX14 4RN

Routledge is an imprint of the Taylor & Francis Group, an informa business

Library of Congress Cataloging-in-Publication Data
Names: Samuel, Kendall Ryndak, author.
Title: Talk behavior to me : the Routledge dictionary of the top 150 behavior analytic terms and translations / Kendall Ryndak Samuel, BCBA.
Description: Abingdon, Oxon ; New York, NY : Routledge, 2025. | Includes bibliographical references and index.
Identifiers: LCCN 2024025510 | ISBN 9781032575254 (hardback) | ISBN 9781032575247 (paperback) | ISBN 9781003439776 (ebook)
Subjects: LCSH: Behavioral assessment.
Classification: LCC BF176.5 .S26 2025 | DDC 150.28/7--dc23/eng/20240809
LC record available at https://lccn.loc.gov/2024025510

ISBN: 978-1-032-57525-4 (hbk)
ISBN: 978-1-032-57524-7 (pbk)
ISBN: 978-1-003-43977-6 (ebk)

DOI: 10.4324/9781003439776

Typeset in Galliard
by KnowledgeWorks Global Ltd.

I dedicate this book to my Uncle Mike, who has unconditionally loved and supported me throughout my whole life, as well as caught thousands of my pitches. He showed me how through hard work, consistency, and love, you can have anything you want in life. THIS is the biggest game of the year. I love you, Uncle Mike.

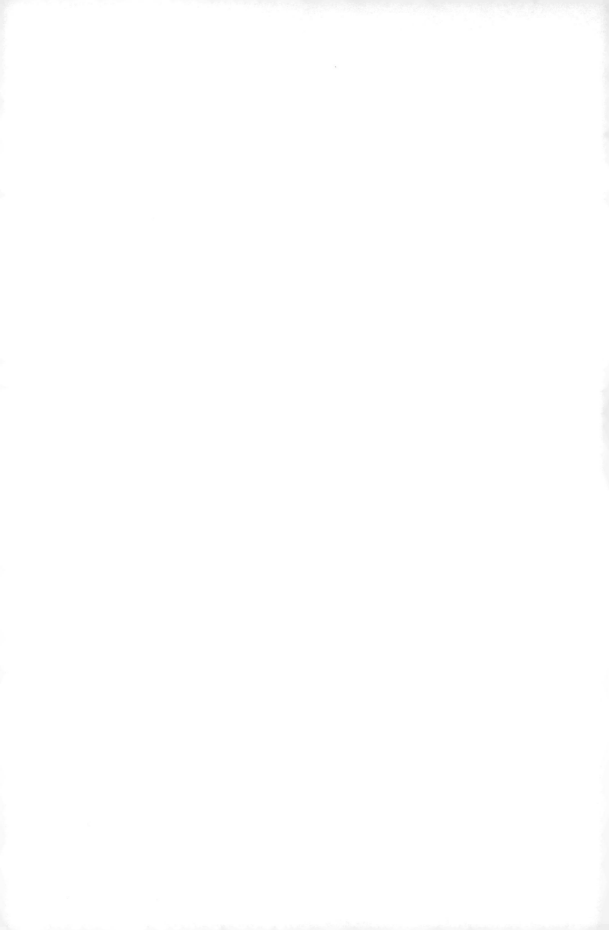

Contents

Figures

Preface

Communication is one of the most foundational skills organisms have. From business partners finalizing deals, orca whales teaching their young how to hunt, and children signing for more hugs, it's everywhere. Using a mutually understood language can make people feel more comfortable with each other and improve the quality of collaboration and problem solving (Noels et al., 1996; Yow & Lim, 2019). I know I'm the happiest when I'm surrounded by people who I feel understand me the best and with whom I can talk freely.

When I first learned about behavior analysis in school, it was like true love at first sight. I was instantly blown away by how this science can explain much of why anything happens in the world (e.g., why my mom chooses the aisle seat on a plane, why you sleep in on Saturdays, why my husband has to have a hotdog when we go to Chicago Cubs baseball games). "Behavior analysis does science very well. It is arguably the most thoroughly rigorous approach to human behavior ever devised" (Vyse, 2013, p. 123). The field has significantly grown and has droves of evidence to show our strategies are extremely effective. Behavior analysis is in an interesting spot though. What is so peculiar is that not many people are even aware that behavior analysis exists. Even with all of the research that has been done and the large amounts of graduate programs, podcasts, YouTube channels, social media pages, and books published, why is behavior analysis still in the shadows?

Practitioners of behavior analysis have mastered communicating with each other, but when it comes to talking with nonbehavior analysts, we don't speak the same language. We use lingo no one has ever heard of before, which is not a great way to market a science that is attempting to expand. The way we speak can come off as intimidating and can further confuse people, decreasing anyone's motivation to listen to what we have to say or use our techniques (Becirevic et al., 2016; Hineline, 1990). We have distanced ourselves from others, including other psychology professionals (Becirevic et al., 2016; Normand, 2014), and we constantly address topics that are unsuccessful at serving broad populations and discuss important issues with jargon that fails to teach and motivate nonbehavior analyst audiences (Becirevic et al., 2016; Friman, 2014; Madden, 2013; Morris, 2014; Pietras et al., 2013; Podlesnik, 2013; Reed, 2014; Schlinger, 2014; St. Peter, 2013; Vyse, 2013, 2014).

For years, behavior analysts have been using language other people don't understand (Critchfield, 2023, September 2). Schlinger (2014) and Morris (2014) stated that one of the best ways to advance behavior analysis is to communicate directly with colleagues outside of our science. Researchers have been suggesting for decades that a second set of everyday terms needs to be created in order to replace technical jargon and improve the spread of accurate behavior analysis information (Bailey, 1991; Lindsley, 1991; Marshall,

2021; Neuman, 2018). *Talk Behavior to Me: The Routledge Dictionary of the Top 150 Behavior Analytic Terms and Translations* was created to help ease the communication about applied behavior analysis between practitioners and others (e.g., technicians, consumers, and other stakeholders). This book may be used in many different ways, including: as a glossary to understand behavior analytic terminology in a more basic way, to translate behavior analytic jargon into simpler terms and phrases, to train future and current behavior analytic practitioners how to communicate with stakeholders about behavior analysis, and for consumers of behavior analytic services to translate their consultant's language.

Each chapter includes behavior analytic terms with at least one translation and two examples. A large number of terms can be found in the books *Applied Behavior Analysis* by Cooper et al. (2020) and *The ABA Visual Glossary* by Shibutani (2022). Additionally, some of the terms have been derived from the book *Verbal Behavior* by B.F. Skinner (1957). Also imbedded into the chapters are details about my time as a behavior analyst, as well as supporting information from other experts in the field on the importance of using basic language when disseminating behavior science. All examples for the terms are derived from different subspecialties in behavior analysis, as well as naturally occurring life events. When teaching others how to communicate using these translations, mentors should individualize how the content is taught to their learners. It is recommended that you determine the learner's current level of competency using this language and create specific goals for the learner based on the skills demonstrated. Let's talk behavior!

References

Bailey, J. S. (1991). Marketing behavior analysis requires different talk. *Journal of Applied Behavior Analysis, 24*(3), 445–448. https://doi.org/10.1901/jaba.1991.24-445

Becirevic, A., Critchfield, T. S., & Reed, D. D. (2016). On the social acceptability of behavior analytic terms: Crowdsourced comparisons of lay and technical language. *The Behavior Analyst, 39*(2), 305–317. https://doi.org/10.1007/s40614-016-0067-4

Cooper, J. O., Heron, T. E., & Heward, W. L. (eds.). (2020). *Applied behavior analysis* (3rd ed.). Merrill Prentice Hall.

Critchfield, T. S. (2023, September 2). 2022's greatest hits of dissemination impact: Insights from the most-noticed articles in behavior analysis. *Association for Behavior Analysis International.* https://science.abainternational.org/2023/09/02/2022s-greatest-hits-of-dissemination-impact-insights-from-the-most-noticed-articles-in-behavior-analysis/

Friman, P. C. (2014). Publishing in journals outside the box: Attaining mainstream prominence requires demonstrations of mainstream relevance. *The Behavior Analyst, 37*(2), 73–76. https://doi.org/10.1007/s40614-014-0014-1

Hineline, P. N. (1990). *Priorities and strategies for this new decade.* Presidential address at the meeting of the Association for Behavior Analysis, Nashville, TN.

Lindsley, O. R. (1991). From technical jargon to plain English for application. *Journal of Applied Behavior Analysis, 24*(3), 449–458. https://doi.org/10.1901/jaba.1991.24-449

Madden, G. J. (2013). Go forth and be variable. *The Behavior Analyst, 36*(1), 137–143. https://doi.org/10.1007/BF03392296

Marshall, K. B. (2021). *The impact of behavior analysis jargon on the effective training of stakeholders* [Doctoral dissertation, Endicott College]. ProQuest. https://www.proquest.com/docview/2571066257?pq-origsite=gscholar&fromopenview=true

Morris, E. K. (2014). Stop preaching to the choir, publish outside the box: A discussion. *The Behavior Analyst, 37*(2), 87–94. https://doi.org/10.1007/s40614-014-0011-4

Normand, M. P. (2014). Opening Skinner's box: An introduction. *The Behavior Analyst, 37*(2), 67–68. https://doi.org/10.1007/s40614-014-0016-z

Neuman, P. (2018). Vernacular selection: What to say and when to say it. *The Analysis of Verbal Behavior, 34*(1–2), 62–78. https://doi.org/10.1007/s40616-018-0097-y

Noels, K. A., Pon, G., & Clement, R. W. (1996). Language, identity, and adjustment. *Journal of Language and Social Psychology, 15*(3), 246–264. https://doi.org/10.1177/0261927x960 153003

Pietras, C. J., Reilly, M. P., & Jacobs, E. A. (2013). Moving forward without changing course. *The Behavior Analyst, 36*(1), 145–149. https://doi.org/10.1007/BF03392297

Podlesnik, C. A. (2013). The openness is there. *The Behavior Analyst, 36*(1), 151–153. https://doi.org/10.1007/BF03392298

Reed, D. D. (2014). Determining how, when, and whether you should publish outside the box: Sober advice for early career behavior analysts. *The Behavior Analyst, 37*(2), 83–86. https://doi.org/10.1007/s40614-014-0012-3

Schlinger, H. D. Jr. (2014). Publishing outside the box: Unforeseen dividends of talking to strangers. *The Behavior Analyst, 37*(2), 77–81. https://doi.org/10.1007/s40614-014-0010-5

Shibutani, M. (2022). *The ABA visual glossary: Applied behavior analysis.* Self-published.

Skinner, B. F. (1957). *Verbal behavior.* Prentice-Hall.

St. Peter, C. C. (2013). Changing course through collaboration. *The Behavior Analyst, 36*(1), 155–160. https://doi.org/10.1007/BF03392299

Vyse, S. (2013). Changing course. *The Behavior Analyst, 36*(1), 123–135. https://doi.org/10.1007/BF03392295

Vyse, S. (2014). Publishing outside the box: Popular press books. *The Behavior Analyst, 37*(2), 69–72. https://doi.org/10.1007/s40614-014-0013-2

Yow, W. Q., & Lim, T. Z. M. (2019). Sharing the same languages helps us work better together. *Palgrave Communications, 5*(1), 154. https://doi.org/10.1057/s41599-019-0365-z

Acknowledgements

I would like to express my deepest gratitude to the following individuals who helped turn this dream book into reality:

- To my husband, Jeff, for being the best model of empathy and kindness, bringing me back into the light, having the best vibes, and for showing me how sweet life can be if you just let go.
- To my Mom, Dad, Dale, and the rest of my family and friends for supporting me throughout the entire writing process. Thank you for collaborating with me, tolerating my jargon, and encouraging me to be brave. With your love, anything is possible.
- To Jeff, and my friends Lindsay, Joe, and Mary for helping me make a decision and take a leap of faith on a wonderful Friday filled with many laughs and great margaritas.
- To my late family members: Uncle Billy, Carson, Yakey, Nanny, Gramcracker, and Aunt Rose. Thank you for being such positive influences in mine and our family's lives. You were the inspiration for the characters in this book.
- To my teachers and professors: Melissa Weber MA, BCBA, LBA, Angela Craven BCBA, LBA, Kathleen Owens, BCBA, LBA, Randy Sanders, BCBA, LBA, SLP, and Ms. Roberts. Thank you for teaching me how to understand the finest details of behavior science and for making it fun!
- To Maggie Pavone, PhD, BCBA-D, LBA, IBA for showing me the ropes on how to teach in higher education and for encouraging me to step outside of the typical areas of ABA practice. You made the space safe for me to grow and do what I love.
- To my clients, colleagues, and students who helped me understand how to apply behavior science to life.
- To all of my followers on social media. Thank you for supporting me and my content! I love making you laugh and teaching you about behavior science. It's been one of the most beautiful experiences of my life.
- To my Auntie Arlene. Thank you for sharing all of your knowledge about public health with me. I've learned so much from you and can't wait to work with you more!

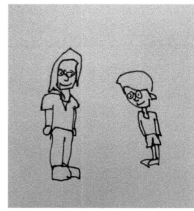

Figure 0.1 "This is an illustration from one of my previous clients. He found much joy in drawing. Thank you for teaching me so much about behavior analysis and life, FM!"

- To softball. You've been with me since the beginning and have set me up for a lifetime of success. Thank you for everything, mi amor. I'm so happy we didn't break up.
- To Dr. Kim Marshall for presenting her dissertation in Boston and for sharing her thoughts on how we can help more people use this brilliant science.
- To Jon S. Bailey, PhD, BCBA-D for giving me the playbook on how to write books, for spending countless hours with me talking about behavior, and for suggesting to the world that we should talk to each other basically about behavior science. That second set of words is finally here!
- To you! Thank you for spending your precious time reading this book. It has been an absolute pleasure creating it for you.

Thank you all for helping me and behavior analysis grow!

About the Author and the Illustrator

Kendall Ryndak Samuel is a board-certified behavior analyst (BCBA) who grew up in Downers Grove, Illinois. She received both her bachelor's and master's degrees from Lindenwood University in St. Charles, Missouri. She is recognized, along with her sister, Dale, in the Downers Grove North High School Hall of Fame for their accomplishments while playing on the school's varsity softball team. She was also a four-year starting softball player and assistant softball coach at Lindenwood University from 2011–2017. Additionally, she has been an adjunct professor and visiting lecturer for Lindenwood University's masters of behavior analysis program. Kendall has worked in various subspecialties of behavior analysis, including dissemination, behavioral sports psychology, organizational behavior management, and autism. She worked with adults and children with autism and other intellectual disabilities from 2016–2023. In 2021, she started two successful social media pages on Instagram and TikTok (@the.behavior.influencer) teaching people about behavior analysis. This led her to winning the Dissemination Board of Behavior Analysis' grant in 2021. She now serves on the Dissemination Board of Behavior Analysis as their Vice President. Last, Kendall is a private softball coach teaching young softball players how to master their skills using behavior analysis. This is Kendall's first book she has published and plans to write more.

John Schuller is an illustrator and educator from Chicago, Illinois. He received his bachelor's degree in fine arts from Loyola University Chicago in 1977 and has done significant work in the art and education industries ever since. John was the illustrator and designer for the Clown Studio in Chicago from 1981–1984, then worked with the Peachtree Studio as a designer and illustrator from 1984–1986. Additionally, John was the illustrator for the book *The Willow Falls Christmas Train*, written by William Trombello. He designed and completed other illustration work in various freelance projects for the Technical Training Corporation too. While playing on his 16-inch softball team in the 1980s, the Pandas, he designed their uniforms and illustrated their logos. John also illustrated logos for other girls fastpitch softball teams in the early 2000s. He has worked as an educator and set designer for Montini Catholic High School and St. Francis High School from 1986–2020.

1 Life Is Never the Same After Studying Behavior Analysis

On the first day of my master's program, my classmates and I were waiting anxiously for our new professor, who, a moment later, flung open the door, threw his bag on the table, scanned the room with his squinted eyes, and declared, "When you finish this class, you'll never think about life the same way again." This put chills down my spine, and he was right. When I finished my first semester, I spoke a different language and *understood* behavior; I could dissect conversations, decode gestures, and even assess the eye contact of others; I felt like I could crack the code. My life had changed. I was hooked on behavior analysis.

Terms and Translations

- **ABC (Antecedent, Behavior, Consequence) Data Recording**
  - **Translation:**
    - Directly observing a behavior and noting what happens directly before and after that behavior.
  - **Examples:**
    - Paul, a behavior analyst, has been asked to find out why a family's dog keeps barking at them when they eat dinner. He observes the family eating and writes down what happens directly before and after the barking.
    - Creed, a behavior analyst, has been asked to find out why employees have been leaving garbage in the breakroom. After observing and tracking what happens before and after trash is left there, he concluded there is no garbage can accessible to the employees in the breakroom.
  - **See:** Antecedent, baseline, behavior, consequence, continuous measurement, and data

- **Abolishing Operation**
  - **Translations:**
    - A phenomenon that makes something less motivating or will make a behavior happen less
    - Making something less desirable or attractive
    - The unmotivator

DOI: 10.4324/9781003439776-1

- **Examples:**

  - Pam's boss tells her, "If you work this weekend event, we will give you a day off." Due to the employee already having unlimited paid time off at the company, this decreases her motivation to work the weekend event.
  - Clara has been experiencing a lot of stress in her life. She usually vents to her friends and family about it, but she can see the venting is starting to negatively affect her relationships. Clara decides to start seeing a therapist to talk through her stress. As soon as Clara started to go to therapy, her motivation decreased to vent to her friends and family since she now vents to her therapist once per week.

- **See:** Conditioned motivating operation, establishing operation, motivating operation, and unconditioned motivating operation

- **Access Maintained Behaviors**

  - **Translations:**

    - Behaving to gain something you want
    - An action that gets you something you value

  - **Examples:**

    - Kim sees all of her friends reading a new book series about romance and fairies. Kim orders the entire series online so she can read it too.
    - Jenny logs her weight loss progress on her app so she can earn rewards.

  - **See:** Positive reinforcement

- **Adjunctive Behavior**

  - **Translations:**

    - An activity to keep you busy
    - Something to do while you wait
    - Time filler behavior/activities
    - Time killers

  - **Examples:**

    - Doodling when sitting at your desk
    - Scrolling on social media while waiting for your doctor's appointment

  - **See:** Behavior

- **Antecedent**

  - **Translations:**

    - An environmental change that happened right before someone responded
    - What happens immediately before a behavior occurs
    - The five seconds before a behavior happens

  - **Examples:**

    - When testing the responses of the robot, James turned on the lights. The robot then looked up at the ceiling. The lights turning on was the antecedent, and the robot looking up was the behavior.

- Right before PJ started to cry, she received an email stating she had won the lottery. The antecedent to PJ crying was receiving the email about the lottery win.

- **See:** Behavior and consequence

- **Antecedent Intervention**

  - **Translations:**

    - Prevention strategies
    - Proactive strategies
    - Strategies to change a potential behavior before it happens

  - **Examples:**

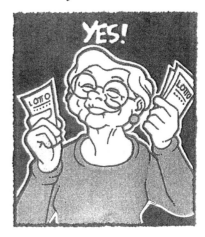

Figure 1.1 "That gratification you hope to experience when you buy lottery tickets."

  - Behavior analysts working for the public health department want to increase how often people clean their hands while in public places. They place hand sanitizer stations throughout every park in a downtown area with a sign that says, "Sanitize your hands before you enter the park and after you leave. Thank you!"
  - At a hotel, putting the towel bin next to the pool exit door to make it more likely for people to throw their towels in the bin instead of on the floor.

  - **See:** Antecedent, functional communication training, high-probability behavior, intervention, non-contingent reinforcement, and proactive.

- **Applied Behavior Analysis (ABA):**

  - **Translations:**

    - The science of analyzing, understanding, and changing behavior.
    - The science of analyzing how the environment affects behavior and how to change it.
    - The science of decision-making, motivation, and teaching habits/skills.
    - Performance management
    - Performance Analysis
    - Behavior modification[1]

  - **Examples:**

    - "The Tree Example": Psychology is like a big tree, which has many branches (e.g., counseling, sports psychology, research, and social work). ABA is one of those branches. ABA has branches underneath it, as well, such as animal behavior, autism and intellectual disabilities, clinical behavior analysis, forensic/crime, health/sports, organizational behavior management, public health behavior analysis, and many others.

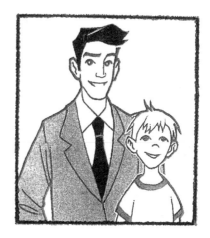

Figure 1.2 "Behavior analysts can work in many different subspecialties, such as child maltreatment prevention."

- Billy is an assistant behavior analyst who uses behavior science to prevent child maltreatment.

- **See:** Behavior, behavior plan, motivating operation, and program

- **Automatic Punishment**

  - **Translations:**

    - Natural punishment
    - Natural occurring events that decrease future behavior
    - Physical discomfort
    - Something that decreases your behavior not involving other people

  - **Examples:**

    - You're lying in bed at night scrolling on your phone. You hold your phone above your face and it drops on your nose and mouth. You then get a fat lip and your face starts to throb. The next time you get in bed, you lay on your side with your phone resting on the bed instead of above your head, so you avoid dropping your phone on your face again.
    - You turn the water on to wash your hands and turn the knob too far to the left. The water scalds your hand. The next time you wash your hands, you make sure to only turn the knob slightly to the left so you avoid scalding your hand again.

  - **See:** Automatic reinforcement and punishment

- **Automatic Reinforcement**

  - **Translations:**

    - Natural reinforcement
    - Natural rewards that increase future behavior
    - Physical pleasure
    - Something that increases your behavior not involving other people

  - **Examples:**

    - Scratching a bug bite to relieve the feeling of the itch
    - The smell of your favorite perfume or cologne

  - **See:** Automatic punishment and reinforcement

- **Aversive Stimulus:**

  - **Translations:**

    - Something unpleasant
    - Something you don't like (e.g., person, place, smell, and taste)

  - **Examples:**

    - Rose does not like to hold cold items, such as a chilled water bottle, a frozen carton of ice cream, or snowballs.
    - Some people cringe when they hear the word "moist."

- **See:** Negative punishment, negative reinforcement, and stimulus

- **Avoidance Contingency**

  - **Translations:**

    - A behavior that prevents or postpones an event from occurring
    - Avoiding events, items, or people you don't like
    - Prevention behavior

  - **Examples:**

    - Putting on deodorant to avoid smelling bad
    - Requiring clean background checks of individuals who want to buy guns to avoid criminals having access to them

  - **See:** Antecedent intervention, aversive stimulus, behavior, contingency, and negative reinforcement

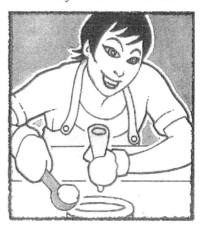

Figure 1.3 "When you don't like to touch cold things, also known as an aversive stimulus, gloves are clutch."

Note

1 This definition can be altered depending on audience, specialty/area of practice, or target behavior(s).

2   Social Media Success

Three years into my career, many changes abruptly occurred. The COVID-19 pandemic made its grand appearance and the world as we knew it would be altered forever. This had a great impact on my career too. I was unhappy and realized I wanted to make a shift to start focusing on professional endeavors I was extremely passionate about. I also wanted to make a difference in behavior analysis but wasn't sure where to turn. During this time, I came across so many people who told me they were confused by the language behavior analysts used and didn't fully understand what we did. Then, I was struck with an overload of inspiration. At the time, I posted about the American TV show, *The Bachelor*, on my Instagram page and loved making people laugh on social media. My dad noticed I loved posting, so he suggested I start teaching my followers about behavior analysis. My heart sang, sparks flew, and I knew this was it. Bridging the gap between behavior analysis and the wider community could be my calling. I saw an opportunity to not only pursue my passions but also to educate and empower others about the transformative power of behavior science. With newfound clarity, I embarked on a journey to redefine my career path, determined to make a meaningful impact both within and beyond the field of behavior analysis.

In June 2021, I made my first post on Instagram, then added it to TikTok soon after. Within five months, I acquired almost 70,000 followers on TikTok with multiple posts gaining over 1 million views. In about three years, my TikTok page has about 82,000 followers and Instagram is nearing 1,000 followers. This speaks to the impact that is possible when behavior analysts use simple language to disseminate our science. Behavior analysts can reach large audiences and teach people how to use our life-changing techniques. We just have to make it accessible to others.

Terms and Translations

- **Backup Reinforcers**
  - **Translations:**
    - Token rewards
    - Secondary rewards
    - Items or activities that are purchased
    - Rewards purchased with money or tokens

DOI: 10.4324/9781003439776-2

- **Examples:**
  - Coach Christy has been giving pitching lessons to local, young softball players for the past ten years. She has saved up enough money to purchase backup reinforcers, such as paying for her wedding and honeymoon.
  - Allee goes to an arcade with her friends. She wins 1,000 tickets, so she purchases some items (backup reinforcers) from the front desk, which were a giant stuffed animal, an arcade gift card, and an iPhone case.

- **See:** Reinforcement and token economy

- **Backward Chaining**

  - **Translations:**

    - Learning the last step of a routine, first.
    - Teaching all steps of a skill, then rewarding the learner for performing the last step. Once they are independent performing the last step, the teacher will then reward them for performing the last two steps of the skill, independently, and so on until the learner is able to perform all steps on their own.

  - **Examples:**

    - A bartender is teaching her newly hired server to make a "Dirty Shirley" drink. The bartender shows the server the following steps:

      - Grab a glass.
      - Put ice in the glass.
      - Pour in two shots of vodka.
      - Pour in lemon lime soda almost all of the way to the top of the glass.
      - Pour in one shot of grenadine.

        - On the last step, the bartender would normally top off the rest of the drink with a spritz of soda. The new server performs this step on his own. The bartender then praises him after he puts in the right amount of soda. Cheers!

    - Patty teaches her cheerleaders their new competition routine. She starts by teaching them the last move first. She rewards them for performing this step correctly, then teaches them the second to last step. Patty rewards them for performing both steps correctly together and follows this exact sequence until the team can perform the entire routine flawlessly.

  - **See:** Backward chaining with leaps ahead, behavior, behavior chain, behavior chain interruption strategy, behavior chain with limited hold, chaining, forward chaining, task analysis, and total task chaining

- **Baseline**

  - **Translations:**

    - Initial phase where the teacher/coach studies the learner's skill(s) without correcting any mistakes or giving feedback.

- Taking data on a learner's skill/behavior without teaching/coaching.
- Testing a behavior without intervening, teaching, or coaching.

- **Examples:**

  - Before putting any changes in place, the police department took data on how many drive-by shootings occurred in a single neighborhood. This would be their baseline data.
  - Before making a treatment plan for her client who is experiencing challenging behaviors due to his depression, Carson tracks to see how long her client lays in bed each day for about two weeks. This is Carson's baseline data that she has collected.

- **See:** Behavior, generalization, intervention, and maintenance

- **Behavior**

  - **Translations:**

    - Actions of living organisms
    - Anything a deceased organism cannot do
    - Habit
    - Response
    - Routine
    - Skill

  - **Examples:**

    - Lynn accidentally sending her grandkids a text that says, "Good Morning!" in the afternoon.
    - Bill kissing his boyfriend.

  - **See:** Access maintained behaviors, adjunctive behavior, behavior chain, escape-maintained behavior, respondent behavior, rule governed behavior, and target behavior

- **Behavior Chain**

  - **Translations:**

    - Habit sequence
    - Habit stacking (Clear, 2018)
    - A sequence of actions. Each action signals the next to occur and makes it more likely for the next action to happen.

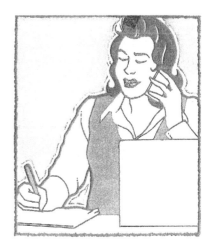

Figure 2.1 "BCBAs can collect data by directly observing a behavior occur or they can receive data indirectly, such as talking to someone over the phone."

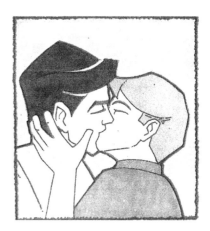

Figure 2.2 "Couples engage in many behaviors together, such as going on dates, asking the other partner if they closed the garage door before leaving the house, and kissing."

- **Examples:**

  - James wanted to teach himself a new morning routine. He started by rewarding himself for getting up and making his bed. Then he rewarded himself for getting up, making his bed, and then eating a healthy breakfast. He ultimately worked his way up to rewarding himself for: getting up, making his bed, eating a healthy breakfast, lifting weights, and then going on a nature walk. Each step signals the next thing to happen.
  - When an emergency operator receives a call, they demonstrate the following steps: ask the caller a series of questions to determine the severity of the emergency, verify the caller's location, dispatch the appropriate emergency responders to the location of the situation, provide the caller with the necessary steps on how to handle the situation, and continue communications with the caller until the emergency responders arrive on the scene. Each step signals the next thing to happen.

- **See:** Backward chaining, backward chaining with leaps ahead, behavior, behavior chain interruption strategy, behavior chain with limited hold, chaining, forward chaining, task analysis, and total task chaining

- **Behavior Chain Interruption Strategy**

  - **Translation:**

    - Pausing someone while they are demonstrating a routine to test if they can finish the rest of it on their own.

  - **Examples:**

    - Angela is working with her elderly client, Debbie, to help her remember to take her medication daily. At 8 am, Angela observes Debbie, which is the time Debbie is supposed to take her medication. Angela starts to talk to Debbie about her plans for the day to test to see if she can remember to take the medication after the conversation. Debbie needed a reminder, so Angela helped her retrieve her pill bottles.
    - Marilyn is teaching her granddaughter, Melanie, to read. Marilyn and Melanie read the words to the book, *Sweet Dream Pie*, together. To see if Melanie can read the rest of the words by herself, Marilyn pauses in the middle of a page, and Melanie reads the rest of the page herself. Good job, Mel!

  - **See:** Backward chaining, backward chaining with leaps ahead, behavior, behavior chain, behavior chain with limited hold, chaining, forward chaining, task analysis, and total task chaining

- **Behavior Chain with Limited Hold**

  - **Translation:**

    - A task/routine must be completed in "x" amount of time before a reward.

  - **Examples:**

    - Mrs. Barnick needs to finish writing her lesson plans by Friday before she can start binge-watching her favorite Hallmark movies all weekend.
    - Harper must finish folding the laundry and cleaning her room before Sunday night in order to earn her allowance.

- **See:** Backward chaining, backward chaining with leaps ahead, behavior, behavior chain, behavior chain interruption strategy, chaining, forward chaining, task analysis, and total task chaining

- **Behavior Plan**

  - **Translations:**

    - A plan to change a behavior, which includes goals and behavior change strategies
    - Coaching plan
    - Curriculum
    - Incentive plan
    - Performance improvement plan
    - Performance plan
    - Teaching plan
    - Training curriculum
    - Training plan

  - **Examples:**

    - Rix is a behavior analyst who works with individuals who are overcoming substance abuse. She puts together a behavior plan for her clients, which includes the following:

      - Assessment of behaviors
      - Behaviors to increase
      - Behaviors to decrease
      - Goals
      - How to react to undesirable behavior
      - How to track all behaviors
      - Incentive/reward system
      - Proactive strategies

    - The government wants to increase the number of electric vehicles being driven to help the health of the environment. The environmental sustainability group hires behavior analysts to create incentive plans to make it more appealing for the country's residents to purchase these vehicles.

  - **See:** Antecedent intervention, intervention, proactive, and reactive

- **Behavior Trap**

  - **Translation:**

    - When an action is easy to do, highly rewarding, but difficult to stop.

  - **Examples:**

    - Sitting with the entire bag of chips and box of fruit rollups next to me when I'm watching a movie. The snacks are irresistible, taste amazing, and are easy to get. I just keep eating them and it's extremely hard to stop.
    - Jason is supposed to be studying for his Spanish test tomorrow. One of his friends sends him a few TikTok videos. Jason ends up watching the video and staying on the app for another 30 minutes. Due to the ease of scrolling, the short duration

of videos, and the algorithm tailoring all of the content on Jason's main screen to his likes, this is a behavior trap.

- **See:** Behavior and reinforcement

- **Behavioral Contrast**

  - **Translations:**

    - Engaging in a behavior more when you are being rewarded more often in one environment or with one person than another.
    - Engaging in a behavior less when you are being rewarded less often in one environment or with one person than another.

  - **Examples:**

    - Carson has two supervisors at her workplace, Holly and Ashley. She emails both of them at least two questions per week about her assigned tasks. Ashley does not respond as quickly to Carson's emails or sometimes at all, but Holly responds within one day. Carson has now begun emailing Holly twice as much during the week instead of emailing Ashley.
    - Blueberry, the dog, barks more for food when he is at his parents' house than when he is at my house because he is given more table food at his parents' house.

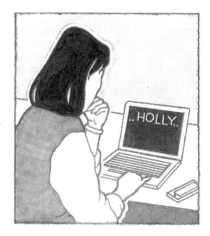

Figure 2.3 "Choosing to email the supervisor who gets back to you in a timely fashion over the one who rarely gets back to you is also known as behavioral contrast."

  - **See:** Behavior, extinction, and reinforcement

- **Behavioral Cusp**

  - **Translation:**

    - A behavior that opens a person up to new rewards, places, people, things, etc.

  - **Examples:**

    - Stacy teaches Rose how to drive. Now that Rose can drive, she can go see her friends downtown that she wasn't able to see much before and go on road trips. Beep Beep!
    - Rachel teaches Smith how to read. Now, he is able to read new books, talk about words he sees on TV with his family, and become a talented author later on in life.

  - **See:** Behavior, pivotal behavior, and reinforcement

- **Behavioral Momentum**

  - **Translation:**

    - Engaging in one action makes it more likely for you to keep engaging in similar actions at a steady rate.

- **Examples:**

  - Jake doesn't typically workout during the week, but he wants to start. He sets a small goal to workout once per week. This becomes easy for Jake, so he starts to work out three times per week, sometimes four.
  - When writing this book, I set a goal for myself to write translations and examples for at least one word per day to make sure I made steady progress. Because I had so much fun writing, I usually would complete two or three words in a day, sometimes more.

- **See:** Behavior and high-probability behavior

- **Behavioral Skills Training (BST)**

  - **Translation:**

    - A teaching strategy using instructions, modeling, rehearsal, and feedback.
    - "Tell-show-do" teaching (Lerman, 2023, p. 3).

  - **Examples:**

    - When teaching his fieldwork student how to write SMART goals, Reese used the following procedure:

      - Explaining the exact format of a SMART goal, why these goals are good to use, and what goals should be focused on first.
      - Reese showed his students examples of how to write these goals.
      - Reese had his student practice writing these goals while he was supervising the student and gave the student feedback.
      - Reese's student then wrote goals for one of his clients, then received feedback from him on her work.

    - Daisy is a social media coach and has been tasked by her client to help teach him how to post a video to social media. She uses the following teaching procedure:

      - Daisy explains the necessary steps on how to make a social media video and post it.
      - Daisy shows her client how she would make a social media video and how to post it.

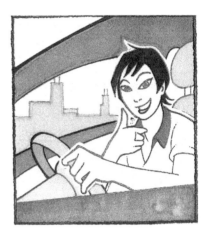

Figure 2.4 "Having a license opens you up to so many fun possibilities in life, such as driving to see your friends, feeling more independent, and taking yourself to your favorite places."

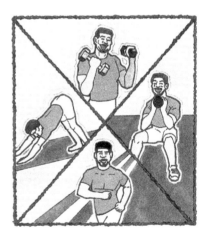

Figure 2.5 "Continuing to exercise regularly can make it more likely for you to keep up with this habit."

- Daisy has her client practice creating videos while she supervises him, then gives him feedback.
- Daisy's client then made a video on his own, posted it, and then she gave him feedback for future posts.

- See: Behavior, behavior plan, and program

- **Board-Certified Assistant Behavior Analyst (BCaBA)**

  - **Translation:**

    - A professional who has earned an undergraduate degree, has completed the necessary coursework and hours in a behavior analysis program, and has passed their boards exam with the Behavior Analyst Certification Board (BACB). They are trained to analyze and change significant behavior. This professional is also able to supervise registered behavior technicians (RBTs) but must practice under the supervision of a board-certified behavior analyst (BCBA).

  - **Examples:**

    - Chester wants to get back into shape but needs help finding the motivation to start working out. He contacts an agency that assigns Chester to a BCaBA, Ernest, to assist him in his fitness journey. After assessing Chester and collaborating with his supervisor, Ernest creates a behavior plan for Chester and consults with his supervising BCBA, Scott, to ensure he is making the correct treatment decisions for Chester.
    - Melissa notices her three-year-old son is still not talking and is engaging in biting himself when he does not get his way. Melissa contacts an agency and is paired with an assistant behavior analyst to help her son learn how to communicate and to help replace his challenging behaviors.

  - **See:** Board-certified behavior analyst and registered behavior technician

- **Board-Certified Behavior Analyst (BCBA)**

  - **Translation:**

    - A graduate-level professional who has earned a masters, specialist, or doctoral degree in behavior analysis. They have also been certified by the BACB. This individual is trained to analyze and change significant behavior. This professional is also able to practice independently (not needing supervision) who is able to supervise BCaBAs and RBTs.

  - **Example:**

    - Marie has developed the habit of forgetting to wear her nightguard to bed. Her dentist is concerned about how badly her teeth grinding has become, so the dentist recommended Marie to see a BCBA to help her develop the habit of wearing her nightguard to bed.
    - A government agency has been called upon to help decrease the number of human trafficking incidents in the United States. They hire BCBAs to help decrease the occurrence of these crimes.

  - **See:** Board-certified assistant behavior analyst and registered behavior technician

References

Clear, J. (2018) *Atomic habits: An easy and proven way to build good habits and break bad ones.* Avery, an imprint of Penguin Random House.

Lerman, D. C. (2023). Putting the power of behavior analysis in the hands of nonbehavioral professionals: Toward a blueprint for dissemination. *Journal of Applied Behavior Analysis, 57*(1), 1–16. https://doi.org/10.1002/jaba.1036

3 Keep It Simple

Behavior analysts have had a history of making explanations about the science more complicated than they need to be. I've observed this during my career and have been guilty of it myself. This can have many negative effects on anyone receiving behavior analytic services, including confusion about the service being provided, incorrect implementation of behavior treatments, a decrease in the effectiveness of plans, and more (Foxx, 1996; Jarmolowicz et al., 2008; Marshall, 2021). Our desire for precision in language and discourse has also led to people perceiving behavior analysts as arrogant and abrasive (Foxx, 1996).

Another effect, which has yet to be studied, is the narrow practice of behavior analysis. Often when I say I'm a behavior analyst, people either ask if I'm a counselor, social worker, or simply assume I work in a school with young children who don't follow the rules. Similar to medicine, there are many branches of behavior analysis. Some examples include acceptance and commitment therapy, applied animal behavior analysis, autism and other developmental disabilities, behavior analysis in military and veterans' issues, behavioral gerontology, behavioral medicine, behavioral pediatrics, behavioral sports psychology, brain injury rehabilitation, child maltreatment intervention and prevention, clinical behavior analysis, education, environmental sustainability, forensic behavior analysis, health and fitness behavior analysis, public health, robotics, organizational behavior management, substance use disorders, and more (Association for Behavior Analysis International, [ABAI] 2023; Behavior Analyst Certification Board [BACB], 2020). Although there are a wide variety of specialties within science, currently, paid job opportunities are slim for behavior analysts outside of working with individuals who have autism or in schools. "We invest so much of our discipline's intellectual capital that affect a relative few" (Critchfield, 2023, September 2, p. 1). I believe one of the reasons for this issue is due to our inability to communicate successfully with people about what we do. We say we can help so many people and have the answers to numerous world issues, but we seem to actively prevent the world from seeing the power of our science (Critchfield, 2023, September 2).

The science was not created to only be used in one area or with one population. "Behavior analysis was meant to be used by citizens of every type" (Bailey, 1991, p. 445). Everyone would be better off if they understood the basics of behavior science and were able to use these strategies on a daily basis to improve their quality of life and that of those around them (Bailey, 1991). Coaches would know how to more effectively motivate their athletes to succeed instead of relying on making them do sprints if they drop a ball. Parents could avoid their child's tantrums by teaching them how to say, "I want down," instead of the child screaming at the top of their lungs until their

DOI: 10.4324/9781003439776-3

father puts them down. You would stop hearing managers say, "My employees only work when I'm around or when I tell them what to do." Many common issues could be avoided if people knew how to use the basics of behavior analysis. People would feel more empowered and have more swagger walking through life because this science gives you the edge.

If the end goal is for the general public to use behavior analysis and for the science to grow its practice, practitioners need to speak basically and make explanations simple so the strategies are accessible for everyone (Marshall, 2021). "A technology has only technical jargon, but … a profession has both technical jargon and a set of plain English equivalents. The development of accurate, comfortable application names may be one of the most important steps in moving from a technology to a profession" (Becirevic et al., 2016, p. 314; Lindsley, 1991, p. 450).

Terms and Translations

- **Chaining**
  - **Translations:**
    - Behavior stacking
    - Habit stacking (Clear, 2018)
    - Linking multiple actions together to create a new routine by rewarding each step, individually, then linking those steps together
  - **Examples:**
    - Jake taught his dog, Blue, to grab his leash and sit by the door before going outside. These were the following steps:
      - Walking to the leash
      - Grabbing the leash with his mouth
      - Walking the leash to the door
      - Hitting the bells on the door with his paw
      - Dropping the leash onto the floor
        - Jake had Blue next to him during all steps of the routine and prompted Blue to demonstrate the last step on his own. Blue was then given a treat when he dropped the leash. Over time, Jake expected Blue to complete more of the steps on his own before eating a treat. After Blue was able to complete all steps of the routine on his own, Blue only received a treat after all steps were completed.
    - At a United States police academy, the trainer taught all of the future officers how to read a person their Miranda Rights. She had all of her students chain together the following statements:
      - You have the right to remain silent.
      - Anything you say can and will be used against you in a court of law.
      - You have the right to an attorney.
      - If you cannot afford an attorney, one will be provided for you.
      - Do you understand the rights I have just read you?

- With these rights in mind, do you wish to speak to me? (Miranda Warning, 2024)

  - After a student correctly stated the first line of the script, the trainer gave the student a thumbs up, and then she read the rest of the script for the student. Next, the student was expected to recite two lines of the script, independently, before receiving a thumbs up. This procedure continued until the student was able to recite all lines of the script on his/her/their own.

- **See:** Backward chaining, backward chaining with leaps ahead, behavior chain, behavior chain interruption strategy, behavior chain with limited hold, forward chaining, task analysis, and total task chaining

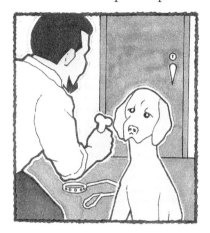

Figure 3.1 "Anyone who performs a series of different actions in a row as a routine has experienced chaining."

- **Classical Conditioning**

  - **Translations:**

    - Training a reflex or automatic response to happen
    - When elements of the environment are presented together over and over again to make the same reflex or response (e.g., being hungry, being tired, sweating, etc.) happen

  - **Examples:**

    - You usually lay in bed when you are tired and are about to go to sleep. You start spraying a lavender scent in the room, night after night, when you lay in bed and are tired. Over time, when you smell lavender outside of your room, you become sleepy.
    - Brooke started a new job! Her new office is freezing, which makes her shiver. One day, the maintenance worker fixes the temperature in the office so it is warmer. Even though the temperature is not cold anymore, Brooke still shivers when she sits down in her office chair.

  - **See:** Automatic reinforcement and operant conditioning

- **Contingency**

  - **Translations:**

    - If you do ____, then you get ____.
    - When a consequence depends on a prior behavior occurring

  - **Examples**

    - In order to improve his independence after a traumatic brain injury, Rodney needed to attend all scheduled therapy sessions.

- Joseph meets a new guy at the bar, Ken. Ken wants Joseph's number. Joseph says he'll give Ken his number, as long as Ken buys Joseph a drink. Smooth.

- **See:** Avoidance contingency

- **Conditioned Motivating Operation**

  - **Translations:**

    - A learned craving
    - Learned motivation
    - An aspect of the environment (e.g., activities, people, places, and objects) that we have learned affects how strong the consequences are and how often a behavior happens

  - **Examples:**

    - In order to increase the amount of account holders at her lingerie company, Naomi has her marketing team send an announcement to their email subscribers stating, "Moving forward, account holders will gain first access to all new products before other customers by signing into your account to shop."

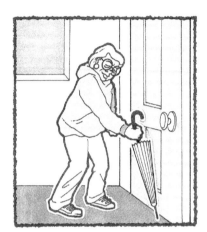

Figure 3.2 "Some of the motivators in your life have been learned over time, such as when the news warns you about possible severe weather or your favorite music artist is coming out with a new album this Friday."

    - PJ is watching the news before she goes to bed. She sees it might rain tomorrow and becomes anxious because she doesn't want to get wet while running her errands. Because she has gotten wet from being in the rain before and wants to avoid the anxiety, she puts her umbrella by the front door so she can take it to work the next day.

  - **See:** Reflexive conditioned motivating operation and transitive conditioned motivating operation

- **Consequence**

  - **Translations:**

    - Ramification
    - Reward
    - Punisher
    - What happens immediately after a behavior/response
    - The result of your actions
    - The result of a behavior

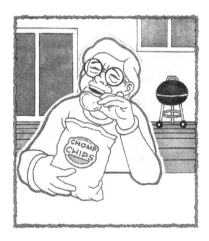

Figure 3.3 "After your stomach growls, you might order a pizza, ask your parents, 'What's for dinner?' or eat some chips."

  - **Examples:**

    - Georgie was driving to see his girlfriend. He was going about 15 miles over the speed limit. A police officer saw this and immediately flipped on his lights and stopped Georgie. The consequence of Georgie speeding was him getting pulled over.

- PJ's stomach growled, so she ate some chips. The consequence of PJ's stomach growling was her eating some chips.

- **See:** Antecedent and behavior

- **Continuous Measurement**

  - **Translations:**

    - Recording all instances of behavior(s)
    - Tracking every time a response happens

  - **Examples:**

    - Jackie tallies every time she buys a box of wine.
    - A dispensary logs every purchase a customer makes of their expensive line of THC gummies.

  - **See:** ABC data recording and discontinuous measurement

- **Continuous Reinforcement**

  - **Translation:**

    - Rewarding a desired behavior every time it happens

  - **Examples:**

    - Christel gives her employees praise every time she sees them helping each other.
    - Parker puts $5 in his vacation savings account every time he finishes a 30-minute workout.

  - **See:** Intermittent reinforcement

- **Correlation**

  - **Translation:**

    - A connection between two events
    - A relationship between two events

  - **Examples:**

    - Frank just got a massage. Now, he feels extremely relaxed. The massage is correlated to how relaxed Frank feels now.
    - The number of times an athlete practices their sport is connected to their success during games or competitions.

- **Count**

  - **Translations:**

    - Tallying
    - Tracking the number of times a response happens

- **Examples:**

  - Taylor tallies how many times her students say, "um," during their speeches.
  - I write down every time I finish a task from my daily planner.

- **See:** Frequency

References

Association for Behavior Analysis International. (2023). *Special interest groups.* Retrieved from https://www.abainternational.org/constituents/special-interests/special-interest-groups.aspx

Bailey, J. S. (1991). Marketing behavior analysis requires different talk. *Journal of Applied Behavior Analysis, 24*(3), 445–448. https://doi.org/10.1901/jaba.1991.24-445

Becirevic, A., Critchfield, T. S., & Reed, D. D. (2016). On the social acceptability of behavior analytic terms: Crowdsourced comparisons of lay and technical language. *The Behavior Analyst, 39*(2), 305–317. https://doi.org/10.1007/s40614-016-0067-4

Behavior Analyst Certification Board. (2023). *Applied behavior analysis subspecialty areas.* Retrieved from https://www.bacb.com/wp-content/uploads/2022/01/Executive-Summary_230412-a.pdf

Clear, J. (2018). *Atomic habits: An easy & proven way to build good habits and break bad ones.* New York, Avery, an imprint of Penguin Random House.

Critchfield, T. S. (2023, September 2). 2022's greatest hits of dissemination impact: Insights from the most-noticed articles in behavior analysis. *Association for behavior analysis international.* https://science.abainternational.org/2023/09/02/2022s-greatest-hits-of-dissemination-impact-insights-from-the-most-noticed-articles-in-behavior-analysis/

Foxx, R. M. (1996). Translating the covenant: The behavior analyst as ambassador and translator. *The Behavior Analyst, 19*(2), 147–161. https://doi.org/10.1007/BF03393162

Jarmolowicz, D. P., Kahng, S., Ingvarsson, E. T., Goysovich, R., Heggemeyer, R., & Gregory, M. K. (2008). Effects of conversational versus technical language on treatment preference and integrity. *Intellectual and Developmental Disabilities, 46*(3), 190–199. https://doi.org/10.1352/2008.46:190-199

Lindsley, O. R. (1991). From technical jargon to plain English for application. *Journal of Applied Behavior Analysis, 24*(3), 449–458. https://doi.org/10.1901/jaba.1991.24-449

Marshall, K. B. (2021). *The Impact of Behavior Analysis Jargon on the Effective Training of Stakeholders* [Doctoral dissertation, Endicott College]. ProQuest. https://www.proquest.com/docview/2571066257?pq-origsite=gscholar&fromopenview=true

Miranda Warning. (2024). *What are your Miranda Rights?* Miranda Warning. http://www.mirandawarning.org/whatareyourmirandarights.html

4   Learning a New Language

When in training to practice behavior analysis, one learns the importance of being able to communicate effectively with clients, stakeholders, and anyone who is not a practicing behavior professional. The extensive involvement of individuals outside of our discipline, such as caregivers, teachers, and other support staff, sets behavior analysis apart from other helping professions (Lerman, 2023). For example, family members are expected to implement reward systems at home and in the community to help their child ask for what they want appropriately. Managers are expected to be consistent with giving employees frequent breaks after a behavior analyst has written this into the plan. The Behavior Analyst Certification Board has an ethical code that states for practitioners to ensure they are using understandable language when communicating with others about behavior analytic services (Behavior Analyst Certification Board [BACB], 2020). While it is emphasized, rarely is the skill formally taught in the classroom or during a student's internship. From my experience, speaking in understandable language was simply talked about. Additionally, most of the practitioners I worked with continued to use heavy jargon in conversations with clients and those with whom we collaborated. I would hear practitioners tell nonbehavior analytic professionals or clients, "More non-contingent reinforcement needs to be implemented into their day," and "We need to increase the response effort in order to abolish their motivation to engage in these problem behaviors." No one outside of our profession knows what they're talking about.

Although speaking basically is an expectation for practitioners, behavior analysts continue to use technical jargon when disseminating their knowledge to others. Lindsley (1991) has been one of the only professionals in behavior analysis' history to attempt to directly translate our language into simpler terms. His work has not gone unnoticed, but unfortunately, a very small amount of practitioners I know are familiar with the article he wrote. This book is an extension of his work.

Terms and Translations

- **Data**
  - **Translation:**
    - The findings
    - The results of what was measured
  - **Examples:**
    - Homeland Security tracks how many attempted and successful terrorist attacks have occurred over the past year in the United States.

DOI: 10.4324/9781003439776-4

- Randy, a behavior analyst, tracks how long it takes his client to start drinking alcohol after a glass of whiskey is put on the kitchen counter.

- **See:** ABC data recording and dependent variable

- **Dependent Group Contingency**

  - **Translation:**

    - One person's behavior determines if the entire group receives a consequence.

  - **Examples:**

    - The manager of a sales team wants everyone to complete their invoices on time. She tells the team, "I am going to pick one person at random. If they get all invoices in on time for the week, we can all leave the office at 1 pm on Friday." Tracy was the employee chosen and she made her goal. The team celebrated at the end of the month by leaving early and getting margaritas. Go Tracy!
    - PJ wants her grandkids to eat all of their vegetables. She tells them, "I'm going to check one of your plates at the end of dinner. If all of the vegetables are eaten, we can all get ice cream." She checked her grandson's plate, and all of the broccoli was gone, so the family celebrated with ice cream cones.

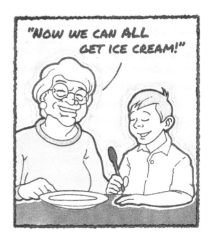

Figure 4.1 "As long as the designated person performs the target behavior correctly, rewards for everyone!"

  - **See:** Group contingency, independent group contingency, and interdependent group contingency

- **Dependent Variable**

  - **Translation:**

    - What is being measured

  - **Examples:**

    - Allie picks her nails a lot during the day. She wants to reduce this, so the first step is to count the number of times she picks her cuticles. The dependent variable is Allie picking her cuticles.
    - The Public Health Department has put a mask mandate in place due to the start of a new pandemic. This will hopefully prevent the population from contracting the new virus. The independent variable is the mask mandate. The dependent variable is the people staying healthy and not contracting the virus.

  - **See:** Independent variable

- **Differential Reinforcement**

  - **Translations:**

    - Rewarding only certain responses
    - When only certain kinds of behavior/habits are rewarded and others are not, usually undesired behaviors.

  - **Examples:**

    - Mrs. Schultz runs the 4th-grade class. She asks the class what they are doing this weekend. She only calls on students to answer who have their hands raised. Mrs. Shultz does not respond to the students who yell out their answers to her.
    - Kat wants a drink from Starbucks. When she goes to pay, the barista says, "Our credit card machine isn't working today, so we are only accepting cash." Kat getting her drink was only rewarded by paying in cash, not with a credit card. If she tries to pay with a card, she will not be given her drink.

  - **See:** Differential reinforcement of alternative behaviors, differential reinforcement of diminishing rates of behavior, differential reinforcement of high rates of behavior, differential reinforcement of incompatible behaviors, differential reinforcement of low rates of behavior, differential reinforcement of other behaviors, negative reinforcement, positive reinforcement, and reinforcement

- **Differential Reinforcement of Alternative Behaviors**

  - **Translations:**

    - Only rewarding a desired behavior that happens for the same reason as the undesired behavior.
    - Rewarding a new behavior, which is replacing a bad habit. Both behaviors happen for the same reason.

  - **Examples:**

    - Erica has a client who is mouthing items in public places (e.g., door knobs and countertops). She ultimately teaches her client to use a chewy, which has the same metallic taste as the public items being mouthed.
    - David's company is having an issue with his employees calling off of work at the last minute. Since his employees were calling off so they could have more time to themselves, David allows them five more days per year of paid time off if they have one or less last-minute call-offs.

  - **See:** Differential reinforcement, differential reinforcement of diminishing rates of behavior, differential reinforcement of high rates of behavior, differential reinforcement of incompatible behaviors, differential reinforcement of low rates of behavior, differential reinforcement of other behaviors, negative reinforcement, positive reinforcement, and reinforcement

- **Differential Reinforcement of Diminishing Rates of Behavior**

  - **Translation:**

    - When a reward is delivered only if a behavior/habit happens less than the criteria. The criteria change over time to lessen how much the behavior/habit occurs.

- **Examples:**

  - Tyler wants to drink less alcohol during the week. He has made a contract with himself that if he only drinks two days during the week, he can go to the bar once on the weekend. He ended up mastering this goal, so he has now set a new goal for himself that if he drinks one day during the week, then he can go to the bars with his friends once on the weekend.
  - Matt is working with a behavior analyst to help him leave the house more and stay at home less. First, he is rewarded for staying at home only six days per week. Then, he is rewarded for only staying at home five days per week.

- **See:** Differential reinforcement, differential reinforcement of alternative behaviors, differential reinforcement of high rates of behavior, differential reinforcement of incompatible behaviors, differential reinforcement of low rates of behavior, differential reinforcement of other behaviors, negative reinforcement, positive reinforcement, and reinforcement

- **Differential Reinforcement of High Rates of Behavior**

  - **Translation:**

    - When a reward is delivered only if the behavior happened more than the criteria.

  - **Examples:**

    - Jackie's daughter, Holly, prefers to use dry shampoo so she doesn't have to wash her hair. Holly hates washing her hair. Jackie tells Holly she will buy her more dry shampoo as long as she washes her hair at least twice per week. Holly is now washing her hair at least three times per week, so Jackie just bought her a new dry shampoo.
    - Anna must log that she attended at least three alcoholics anonymous meetings for one month straight to her behavior analyst before earning her cash reward. Anna attended four meetings during the month, so she earned her reward.

  - **See:** Differential reinforcement, differential reinforcement of alternative behaviors, differential reinforcement of diminishing rates of behavior, differential reinforcement of incompatible behaviors, differential reinforcement of low rates of behavior, differential reinforcement of other behaviors, negative reinforcement, positive reinforcement, and reinforcement

- **Differential Reinforcement of Incompatible Behaviors**

  - **Translation:**

    - Rewarding a behavior that cannot be done at the same time as the undesired behavior.

  - **Examples:**

    - Janet likes to eat a lot of dessert after dinner. When she starts to desire dessert, Janet will go on a walk. She cannot go on a walk outside and eat desserts in her house at the same time. As soon as Janet starts her walk without snacking, she turns on her favorite music playlist.

- Vanessa's toddler tends to put her hands in her diaper when Vanessa changes her. Now, when Vanessa changes her daughter's diaper, she gives her a toy to hold. Vanessa's daughter can't hold the toy and put her hands in her diaper at the same time. After a successful diaper change, Vanessa dances and sings with her daughter.

- **See:** Differential reinforcement, differential reinforcement of alternative behaviors, differential reinforcement of diminishing rates of behavior, differential reinforcement of high rates of behavior, differential reinforcement of low rates of behavior, differential reinforcement of other behaviors, negative reinforcement, positive reinforcement, and reinforcement

- **Differential Reinforcement of Low Rates of Behavior**

  - **Translation:**

    - When a reward is delivered only if the behavior/habit happened less than the expectation. The expectation does not change over time.

  - **Examples:**

    - The US hockey team is practicing for the Olympics. They keep missing shots on goal during their games. Their coach told the team, "If you guys can miss less than two shots during this drill, we can leave practice and go home."
    - Arlene is a behavior analyst who works with individuals who have obsessive-compulsive disorder (OCD). She is currently working with a client to help him only engage in one of his rituals once per day. If he meets his goal, he buys himself something from his Amazon cart.

  - **See:** Differential reinforcement, differential reinforcement of alternative behaviors, differential reinforcement of diminishing rates of behavior, differential reinforcement of high rates of behavior, differential reinforcement of incompatible behaviors, differential reinforcement of other behaviors, negative reinforcement, positive reinforcement, and reinforcement

- **Differential Reinforcement of Other Behaviors**

  - **Translations:**

    - Getting a reward if you do literally anything else except for the undesired behavior.
    - Do anything else but this one thing."

  - **Examples:**

    - Kale's son really wants more time at the pool, but he likes to put pool water in his mouth when he swims. As long as Kale's son doesn't put the pool water in his mouth, even though he was running around the pool and splashing a lot, Kale still rewarded him with extra swimming time.
    - Brent is hired by a family to watch their house during the summer. The family wants him to stay out of the west wing of the home, so they told Brent, "You can go anywhere you want in the house. As long as you don't go into the west wing, you will receive your weekly paycheck. We'll be watching on our cameras."

- **See:** Differential reinforcement, differential reinforcement of alternative behaviors, differential reinforcement of diminishing rates of behavior, differential reinforcement of high rates of behavior, differential reinforcement of incompatible behaviors, differential reinforcement of low rates of behavior, negative reinforcement, positive reinforcement, and reinforcement

- **Direct Measurement**

  - **Translations:**

    - Observing and measuring behavior(s) with your own eyes
    - Being physically present to see a behavior/habit happen

  - **Examples:**

    - John observed customers for his entire shift and wrote down how many people actually signed up for the store's credit card. No one signed up.
    - Peter tallied how many sodas his wife drank on their long road trip.

  - **See:** ABC data recording, count, duration, frequency, interresponse time, latency, and magnitude

- **Discontinuous Measurement**

  - **Translation:**

    - Measuring only certain instances of a behavior but not all.

  - **Examples:**

    - Alyssa is a teacher and wants to increase how often her students help each other while she's tending to others. She sets a timer on her phone to go off every five minutes while she's assisting her students. As the timer starts to chime, she looks to see if any of the students are helping each other. If she sees them offering support to each other, Alyssa cheers for the class and marks a tally in her notebook.
    - Jenny is a clinical director and wants to decrease how much people gossip while they work. When she comes out of her office, she sets a timer on her smart watch. If gossiping happened at all before the timer started to buzz, she writes this down.

  - **See:** Momentary time sampling, partial-interval recording, and whole interval recording

- **Discrete Trial**

  - **Translation:**

    - Practice trials to create a single new habit with clear reminders and consequences.

  - **Examples:**

    - Julie is teaching her new hire, Jessie, how to make a chai tea latte at the coffee shop. Julie first has to teach Jessie what ingredients go into the latte. She sets them out and says, "Jessie, give me one ingredient that goes into the latte." After Jessie hands Julie each correct ingredient, Julie praises Jessie and gives her a check on her progress board.

- Marybeth, a pediatric behavior analyst, is teaching a family how to implement a sleep protocol for their daughter. She first describes all of the correct steps in the protocol. Marybeth then asks a series of questions, "What time should you start your daughter's bedtime routine?" When the family answers, "7 pm," she praises them, then moves onto the next question.

- **See:** Consequence, error correction, incidental teaching, prompt, and reinforcement

- **Discriminative Stimulus**

  - **Translations:**

    - A sign that lets you know what to do or not to do next
    - A signal that lets you know if a reward or punisher is possible
    - An indicator or signal that consistently makes you behave in a certain way
    - "When you sense this, you know to do X."

  - **Examples:**

    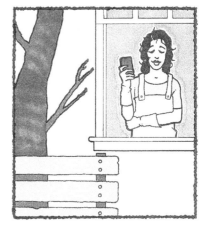

    - A red circle appears on top of the email icon on your phone. You know this means you have an unread email in your inbox, so you click on it. The red circle is the discriminative stimulus for letting you know clicking the email will get you access to something you may possibly want (e.g., new information and a promo code).
    - Carson is trying to complete all of her daily tasks and becomes overwhelmed. She begins having a panic attack. She sees that the bench in front of her pond is open. This reminds her that she can sit and take a short break to relieve some of her anxiety. Woosah.

  - **See:** Reinforcement, punishment, stimulus control, and stimulus

    Figure 4.2 "A signal that lets you know feeling calm is available is very powerful in stressful situations."

- **Duration**

  - **Translation:**

    - How long a behavior/habit happens

  - **Examples:**

    - It took the police six years to catch John Wayne Gacy for murdering his victims. The duration of the police of her anxiety. (The red Berry, **2022**).
    - Leandra takes about 30 minutes to prep and mix all of the ingredients for her famous silver cake; her goal is to get this down to 20 minutes and then she will prepare a YouTube video demo for her fans.

  - **See:** Data and direct measurement

References

Behavior Analyst Certification Board. (2020). *Ethics code for behavior analysts.* https://bacb.com/wp-content/ethics-code-for-behavior-analysts/

Berry, P. A. (2022). *Why serial killer John Wayne Gacy escaped suspicion for so long. https://www.netflix.com/tudum/articles/conversations-with-a-killer-john-wayne-gacy-director-interview*

Lerman, D. C. (2023). Putting the power of behavior analysis in the hands of nonbehavioral professionals: Toward a blueprint for dissemination. *Journal of Applied Behavior Analysis, 57*(1), 1–16. https://doi.org/10.1002/jaba.1036

Lindsley, O. R. (1991). From technical jargon to plain English for application. *Journal of Applied Behavior Analysis, 24*(3), 449–458. https://doi.org/10.1901/jaba.1991.24-449

5   What Kind of Behavior?

From my observations, many people relate the word "behavior" to negative actions: disobeying rules, breaking the law, creating issues, being off task, and many more. When watching a press conference, you'll often hear people say, "We don't tolerate this kind of behavior." Sitting at a restaurant for drinks, you might overhear a group of friends exclaim, "Don't put up with that behavior anymore. Just dump him." Foxx (1996) was not surprised to find from his research that most people found the word "behavior" to be more negative. Popular media has long assumed that behavior analysis focuses on bad behavior rather than all forms of it (Foxx, 1996). As behavior analysts understand it, behavior is anything a living organism can do. If behavior analysts continue to say things like "He had a lot of behaviors today," or, "We're working on her behavior," it continues to pair the word "behavior" with negative events and actions. People will keep assuming we only work to get rid of "bad behavior" or "bad habits." It is a practitioner's duty to change how the world perceives behavior and our science.

When talking about behavior with others, make sure to define exactly what behavior you are talking about so you are using our terminology accurately. This will give the word "behavior" a chance to be paired with every kind of action a living organism can do, not just problematic ones. For example, instead of me saying, "I saw a lot of behaviors at the beach," I could say, "I saw a lot of playful behavior at the beach, like people dancing, playing games, and swimming." Specifying the behavior will help others outside of the behavior analysis field use our terminology accurately. Model the behavior you want to see!

Terms and Translations

- **Echoic**
  - **Translation:**
    - Repeating someone's sounds, words, or phrases
  - **Examples:**
    - Glenn, a motivational speaker, yells to the crowd, "I WANNA HEAR YOU SAY, 'YES I CAN!'" The crowd yells back, "YES I CAN!"
    - A mother is teaching her son how to be polite after someone gives him a gift. After he is handed the gift, his mother says, "Thank you," and he echoes, "thank you."
  - **See:** Verbal behavior

DOI: 10.4324/9781003439776-5

- **Elicit**
  - **Translations:**
    - Drawing out an automatic response or reflex from someone
    - Extracting an unlearned response
  - **Examples:**
    - Cutting an onion made my eyes start to water uncontrollably. The cut onion elicited my "crying."
    - When Lindsay entered the sauna, she immediately started to drip with perspiration.
  - **See:** Emit and evoke

- **Emit**
  - **Translation:**
    - Behaving
    - Engaging in an action
    - Producing a response
  - **Examples:**
    - Jeff proposed to me exactly as my dad asked my mom to marry him. Jeff emitted the response of saying, "Do you want to do this?"
    - In response to recent oil spills, the United States Environmental Protection Agency (EPA) staff posted about the impacts of climate change on our oceans and what we can do to help. The EPA staff emitted the response of alerting our nation about climate change.
  - **See:** Behavior, elicit, and evoke

- **Error Correction**
  - **Translations:**
    - A plan for correcting mistakes
    - How a coach, teacher, or trainer responds to an error their student makes
  - **Examples:**
    - Mr. Parr, a teacher, is reviewing the continents of the world with his class. Instead of saying, "South America," the class said, "South Africa." He pointed to the map and said, "What's the last continent? South America." Then, he asked the class again, "What's the last continent?" The class had to answer the question correctly twice before moving onto the next activity.
    - A behavior analyst is working with a family to help their daughter go to bed on time. The first step for the family is to remind their daughter that it will be time to go upstairs in five minutes. The family tells the behavior analyst that the plan is not working. The behavior analyst finds the family is forgetting the first step of the plan, so she has the family repeat the first step twice before moving on to helping their daughter clean up her toys.
  - **See:** Behavior plan

- **Escape Maintained Behaviors**

  - **Translations:**

    - Getting away from something or someone you don't like.
    - Ways to get someone out of a place, activity, away from a person, or from something they don't like.

  - **Examples:**

    - Kevin is at a house party with his friends, but they're playing terrible music. He wants to leave, so Kevin goes back to his house to binge his favorite show without telling anyone, also known as an Irish goodbye or an escape-maintained behavior.
    - Mittens, a smart puppy, lays in the grass while her mommy waters the flowers on a hot summer day. Once Mittens starts to pant, she gets up and walks to a shady spot under the tree so she can escape the heat and direct sunlight. What a good girl.

  - **See:** Behavior and avoidance contingency

- **Escape Extinction**

  - **Translations:**

    - Preventing leaving a situation
    - Not allowing the removal of an undesired person, place, or thing until a certain expectation is fulfilled.

  - **Examples:**

    - When your parents say, "You can't leave the table until you eat all of your vegetables and drink all of your milk," even though you want nothing more than to leave the kitchen.
    - A group of police bust a college house party. They have the house surrounded and they make an announcement to all of the people inside saying, "No one leaves until we have seen everyone's licenses and student IDs."

  - **See:** Extinction, extinction burst, and spontaneous recovery

- **Establishing operation**

  - **Translation:**

    - A craving that makes something more motivating or will make a behavior happen more.

  - **Examples:**

    - Carson and Mac are in a long-distance relationship and haven't seen each other in four months. This has increased their motivation to spend all weekend together and made alone time very valuable.
    - Smoking marijuana or eating tetrahydrocannabinol (THC) edibles can make snacks extremely sought after due to getting the "munchies." Being high is the

establishing operation for wanting to eat a bunch of snacks because they are so delicious and you become so high.

- **See:** Abolishing operation, conditioned motivating operation, motivating operation, and unconditioned motivating operation

- **Evoke**

  - **Translations:**

    - Drawing out a learned habit/response from someone
    - Extracting a learned response

  - **Examples:**

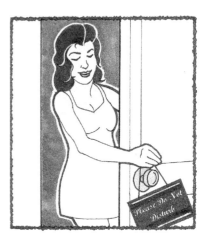

Figure 5.1 "This kind of motivation increases your want for something."

  - The news said the weather was going to be 90 degrees and sunny today. Coach Redmer made sure to wear a hat and sunscreen. The weather update evoked him putting on sunscreen and a hat before he left the house.
  - At my previous job, we conducted family guidance trainings to help families implement treatment plans and prevent child maltreatment. Working with families evoked us to complete family guidance trainings.

  - **See:** Behavior, elicit, and emit

- **Extinction**

  - **Translations:**

    - Not being rewarded for engaging in a behavior anymore
    - Rewards being discontinued for a certain response

  - **Examples:**

    - Kenzie is a toddler and goes to the park with her mom almost every day. It started to rain, so her mom said they would go to the park tomorrow. Stacy not bringing Kenzie to the park is an example of extinction.
    - PJ's grocery store is closed (extinction), so she will not be able to shop (reinforcement/reward) there anymore.

  - **See:** Escape extinction, extinction burst, and spontaneous recovery

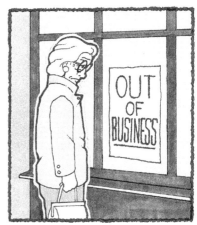

Figure 5.2 "Extinction can come in all forms, such as not receiving attention anymore for yelling out answers in class, a subscription no longer being available to you, or when your favorite store closes."

- **Extinction Burst**

  - **Translations:**

    - An initial spike in how often a behavior happens when it no longer is rewarded
    - When a behavior happens more than it typically does after it is not rewarded anymore

  - **Examples:**

    - Karen is on a flight and pressed the assistance button to ask if she can smoke her e-cigarette on the flight. The flight attendants say, "Absolutely not." Karen does not like this, so she presses the assistance button again to ask if she can just take one puff. The flight crew once again said, "No." Karen presses the button about 20 more times and harder each time, but no one attends to her. Karen's increase in pressing the button after being ignored was an extinction burst.

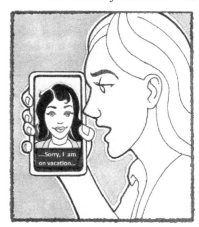

Figure 5.3 "We have all experienced a burst of behavior when we aren't able to access what we want. We'll try and try to get what we want until we either have it or we realize it's not going to happen."

    - Carson is on vacation. Someone wants to get in contact with her, but Carson's phone is off. This person texted Carson twice, then three more times, then tried calling her and leaving her several voicemails. The increase in attempts to contact Carson was an extinction burst.

  - **See:** Escape extinction, extinction, and spontaneous recovery

- **Fixed Interval Schedule of Reinforcement**

  - **Translations:**

    - When a reward is delivered after a set amount of time
    - When you get what you want after a specific amount of time has passed
    - After X amount of time, you get (name of reward).

  - **Examples:**

    - Every Black Friday, or the Friday after Thanksgiving in America, most stores and websites have huge sales. Customers can purchase their favorite items at a reduced cost in many stores and online.
    - Jake is paid every two weeks by his employer.

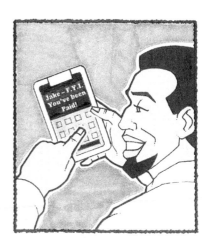

Figure 5.4 "Some rewards, like a paycheck, are delivered after a specific amount of time has occurred."

- **See:** Fixed ratio schedule of reinforcement, variable interval schedule of reinforcement, and variable ratio schedule of reinforcement

- **Fixed Ratio Schedule of Reinforcement**

  - **Translations:**

    - When a reward is delivered after a specific number of responses/actions
    - After X number of (name of action), you get (name of reward).

  - **Examples:**

    - For every video I post to social media, my husband gives me one like. Thanks, Babe!
    - For every one dollar Billy spends at his favorite makeup store, he earns one reward point.

  - **See:** Fixed interval schedule of reinforcement, variable interval schedule of reinforcement, and variable ratio schedule of reinforcement

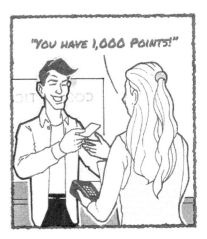

Figure 5.5 "Some rewards, like earning points at your favorite store, are delivered after you've demonstrated a set number of actions, such as buying items."

- **Forward Chaining**

  - **Translation:**

    - Learning the initial step, first of a routine.
    - Rewarding a learner for performing the first step of a routine. Once they are independently performing the first step, the instructor will then reward them for performing the first and second steps of the routine, and so on until the learner is able to perform all steps on their own.

  - **Examples:**

    - My husband was the one who taught me how to pump gas. He started by teaching me the first step, which was to open the cover to the gas tank. He told me, "Good job!" when I did it by myself. He carried out the same procedure as he taught me the rest of the steps. When I tried to learn to pump gas with my mom, I ended up spraying her in the mouth with gas. Sorry, Peach!
    - In the baseball umpire training program, future umpires learn how to call balls and strikes. The trainer teaches all of the students the first step, which is where to stand behind the catcher. They receive praise for doing this correctly. The trainer then teaches the students where to stand and how to bend their knees so they can see the pitches from the correct height, then rewards his students. The trainer follows this procedure until all students can demonstrate the correct steps for standing behind the catcher and calling pitches balls and strikes.

  - **See:** Backward chaining, backward chaining with leaps ahead, behavior chain, behavior chain interruption strategy, behavior chain with limited hold, chaining, forward chaining, task analysis, and total task chaining

- **Frequency**

  - **Translation:**

    - How often something happens

  - **Examples:**

    - Counting how many times I spray my favorite perfume
    - You've been to the same Pilates studio ten times

  - **See:** Data and direct measurement

- **Functional Analysis (FA)**

  - **Translation:**

    - An experiment that tests different conditions to find the definitive answer as to why a behavior/habit is happening. The answers help a behavior analyst make decisions on how to come up with a treatment plan.

  - **Examples:**

    - An individual is engaging in hitting other people, so his practitioners run an analysis to test what makes him engage in this response. They test the following conditions in a clinic: the client having access to all of his favorite items and people, the client being alone, when attention is taken off of him, when demands are placed on him, and when his favorite items are taken from him. The findings from this test help his practitioners understand why hitting keeps occurring and how to create a treatment plan to make the hitting stop.
    - A construction company is having issues with their employees not wearing their hardhats while on site. A behavior analyst is hired to find out why. She tests to see if it is because: (1) people are forgetting them at home, (2) there aren't reminders on site to wear the hardhats, (3) the hardhats are uncomfortable, or (4) if the workers don't understand *why* they have to wear them. She then tests all of these possibilities. The answers from the analysis will help the behavior analyst create a plan to improve safety on the job site.

  - **See:** Behavior, functional behavior assessment, and function of behavior

- **Functional Behavior Assessment (FBA)**

  - **Translation:**

    - An informal assessment that may find out why a behavior/habit is happening. This may include interviews, tracking the behavior, and observations.

  - **Examples:**

    - When starting with a new client or group, a behavior analyst will interview them (if appropriate) and others close to the them to gain information on any challenges they are facing, when they happen, what typically triggers them, and what happens right after these behaviors. This helps the behavior analyst create a treatment plan for their client or group.

- A behavior analyst has been contracted to help the executive team at a big company because they are having a difficult time figuring out why their turnover rate is so high. The behavior analyst schedules observations of the employees and takes data. She also interviews current employees. Both methods help her find the answers she needs in order to come up with a plan to help the company decrease their turnover rate.

- **See:** Behavior, behavior plan, functional analysis, and function of behavior

- **Functional Communication Training**

  - **Translation:**

    - Teaching communication skills to replace challenging behaviors

  - **Examples:**

    - Teaching my parent's dog to ring a bell with his paw to let them know he has to go outside instead of barking at the door or at my parents.
    - A teacher teaches his students to ask for help instead of cheating off of someone's paper or becoming off task during class. When the students ask the teacher for help and refrain from engaging in the undesirable responses, he praises them and offers them the help they need.

  - **See:** Antecedent intervention, function of behavior, and verbal behavior

- **Function of Behavior**

  - **Translation:**

    - The reason why a behavior happens

  - **Examples:**

    - I drink an espresso martini to get a buzz.
    - Mary puts her TV remote away before she leaves so her dog, Papa, doesn't chew on it.

  - **See:** Behavior, functionally equivalent/compatible, functional analysis, functional behavior assessment, and response class

- **Functionally Compatible/Equivalent**

  - **Translations:**

    - Having the same purpose
    - Behaviors happening for the same reason

  - **Examples:**

    - I sing to my favorite songs or meditate to stop my anxious thoughts. Both of these behaviors happen for the same reason, which is to decrease my anxiety.
    - Ted Bundy flirted with women and acted like he needed help by flaunting his fake broken arm in order to lure his victims close enough to him so he could kidnap them. Both of these behaviors happened for the same reason, which was to get access to his next victims.

- **See:** Behavior, function of behavior, and response class

References

Foxx, R. M. (1996). Translating the covenant: The behavior analyst as ambassador and translator. *The Behavior Analyst, 19*(2), 147–161. https://doi.org/10.1007/BF03393162

6   Switch It Up

Researchers have discovered many positive effects derived from practitioners using simpler language. For example, when behavior analysts changed their language to align with more commonly used terms, their methods and strategies were implemented more accurately and used more often (Al-Nasser et al., 2019; Bailey, 1991; Graff & Karsten, 2012; Lindsley, 1991; Marshall, 2021; Smith, 2016). Additionally, Foxx (1996) and Lerman (2023) suggested for behavior analysts to explain why their recommendations are effective by using concepts and terminology related to a specific profession. For instance, behavior analysts should use language spoken among the sports community when working with coaches and athletes. Learning the language of other professionals and organizations and using those terms when speaking to them about using behavior analytic strategies will help our science become more accepted and will help behavior analysts build strong alliances with other professionals (Foxx, 1996; Lerman, 2023). Outside of collaborating with other behavior analysts, we should think of ourselves as behavior science ambassadors and translators (Foxx, 1996).

I experienced more success with my treatment plans being written in basic terminology first-hand when I worked in the clinical setting. For example, when a client would demonstrate a correct response, I used to write notes about what reward to present and how often. When I first started in the field, I would write, "Reinforcement Schedule: Fixed Ratio 1." What I should have written was, "Deliver (name of reward) every time (name of client) does (name of behavior)." Not realizing this at the time, the only people who were able to translate that note were other behavior analysts, who unfortunately were not the ones implementing the plan. The crazy thing is that behavior analysts are rarely the ones who regularly and directly administer these plans and strategies. Consumers and other professionals, such as behavior technicians, families, managers, executives, coaches, and other stakeholders, are the people who typically carry out the plans. So why aren't behavior analysts using language these individuals understand?

I would receive so many questions from people asking me, "What does this mean?" and "Can you explain that to me again?" Even talking to my friends and family about what I do, their faces go blank and their eyes glaze over when I throw in terms like "motivating operation" or "negative reinforcement." Once I started to explain the science using the basic terms included in this book, so many wonderful things happened: the plans I wrote were being implemented more accurately, my social media following grew immensely, and people wanted to listen to what I had to say. The jargon we use is like a foreign language to everyone else outside of science. Behavior analysts need to make sure we use simple terminology when talking with nonbehavior analysts. This will ensure proper usage of our treatment plans and avoid creating negative interactions with others. We must have a

DOI: 10.4324/9781003439776-6

language that is understood and approved by people outside of the field because how others perceive our language shapes how they view our values (Fowler, 1991; Foxx, 1996).

Even if we have the best intentions and tons of research to show how successful our strategies are, if we use words like "manipulation" or "punishment" with the wrong crowd, people may see us as controlling, harsh, or abrasive professionals. "Translation helps broaden the audience" (Foxx, 1996, p. 154). We have a lot to say and can help so many people, but we need to do that in a way that will make people want to listen, not tune us out. This approach can lead to improved collaboration and understanding across disciplines and foster a more cohesive and effective application of behavior analytic principles. By adapting language to suit different contexts, behavior analysts can bridge communication gaps and tailor interventions to better meet the needs of diverse populations. Embracing this flexibility in language can ultimately enhance the impact and reach of behavior analysis in various settings and industries.

Terms and Translations

- **Generalization**

  - **Translations:**

    - When skills or behaviors someone learned occur with multiple people, in multiple places, and in multiple situations
    - When you learn one action and begin doing similar actions that you were not trained to do

  - **Examples:**

    - When Rose was in driver's education, she learned red meant "stop." Now, she knows to stop at traffic lights, stop signs, and when she sees someone's taillights since they are all red.
    - My parents taught me how to pack for a trip by folding my clothes, then putting them in the luggage. I realized I could fit more clothes in my bag by rolling my shirts and pants, then putting them in my luggage.

  - **See:** Response generalization and stimulus generalization

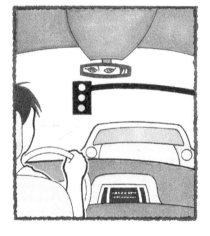

Figure 6.1 "With generalization, you can either attempt a new version of a skills you were taught or respond to different signals in the same way."

- **Group Contingency**

  - **Translation:**

    - A plan to reward or punish a group's behavior

  - **Examples:**

    - My entire college softball team had to run from foul pole to foul pole after a game for the number of strikeouts we had when batting.
    - In order for a department to come back into the office after a pandemic, people had to show proof of their up-to-date vaccine cards.

- **See:** Dependent group contingency, independent group contingency, interdependent group contingency, reinforcement, and punishment

- **Habit Reversal**

  - **Translation:**

    - A behavior change strategy, which includes:

      - Self-awareness
      - Understanding triggers
      - Choosing a behavior to replace your unwanted habit (usually something you cannot do at the same time as the "bad habit")
      - Rewarding your new habit

  - **Examples:**

    - When I decided I wanted to stop biting my nails, I chose to treat this in a variety of steps:

      - Becoming aware of when I bit my nails and what triggered me to do so.
      - Making sure my nails are always done every 3–4 weeks.
      - When I feel triggered, I make sure I use a fidget or sit on my hands.
      - Every time my husband saw me not biting my nails, he would praise me.

    - Julia wants to decrease snacking on unhealthy foods. She followed a habit reversal plan, which included:

      - Being aware of her triggers, which included smoking marijuana and sitting for longer than 10 minutes
      - Keeping unhealthy snacks in inconvenient places in the pantry
      - When she felt triggered, she would drink water or eat vegetables or fruit.
      - Julia rewarded herself every time she refrained from eating an unhealthy snack by putting a check mark on her calendar. Once she reached five check marks, she would make a facial appointment.

  - **See:** Behavior, behavior plan, differential reinforcement of incompatible behaviors, and self-management

- **Habituation**

  - **Translations:**

    - Being less responsive to something in the environment after coming in contact with it over and over again
    - Desensitizing to something in the environment
    - Getting used to something in the environment

  - **Examples:**

    - My husband really wanted me to eat more spicy food with him, so he would slowly add more red pepper flakes to all of the dishes he cooked for us. After about a month of him doing this, I couldn't even taste the spice from the red pepper flakes anymore. Touché, Babe.

- Rose is scared of loud sounds and often avoids certain places and events if she knows there is a chance of them being loud. She works with her behavior analyst to help her get over this fear. Rose's behavior analyst presents her with louder sounds during each of their sessions together over and over again. After many sessions together, Rose has overcome her fear of loud sounds and was able to attend the summer fireworks with her friends this year.

- **See:** Systematic desensitization

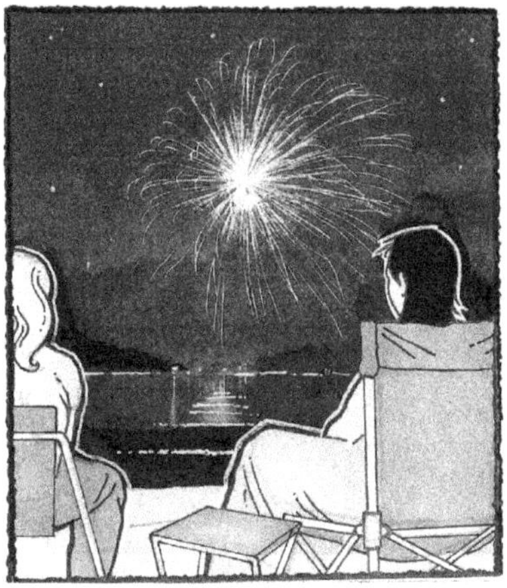

- **High-Probability (High-P) Behavior**

  - **Translation:**

    - An action someone is highly likely to do

  - **Examples:**

    - A group of friends is likely to talk with each other when they sit together in class.
    - When someone says they'd like to make a "toast," people are likely to clink their champagne glasses together and say, "cheers," afterwards.

  - **See:** Antecedent intervention, behavior momentum, and proactive

- **Incidental Teaching**

  - **Translation:**

    - Teaching lessons in real-life situations as they happen

  - **Examples:**

    - A teacher noticed one of her students sitting alone on the playground. The student told her he didn't know how to ask the other students if he could join. The teacher told him what to say. Then, he went up to his classmates and said, "Hey, can I play?"
    - Chris is giving a speech on how to negotiate. His mentor is in the front row and notices Chris is looking down at his notes instead of the crowd. When Chris makes eye contact with his mentor, his mentor gives him a cue to keep his head up while talking.

  - **See:** Classical conditioning, discrete trial, and operant conditioning

- **Independent Group Contingency**

  - **Translation:**

    - Only the people in the group who meet the set criteria earn the reward/ punisher.

Figure 6.2 "One can become less reactive to stimuli in the environment when it is presented over and over again."

- **Examples:**

  - In our circle time group at one of my previous jobs, only the clients who had their hands raised were the ones allowed to answer the questions from the therapist.
  - Only employees at Jake's job who submit their time cards before the due date receive their paychecks.

- **See:** Dependent group contingency, group contingency, and interdependent group contingency

- **Independent Variable**

  - **Translations:**

    - The curriculum
    - The intervention
    - The strategy or strategies
    - The treatment
    - The change you are putting in place

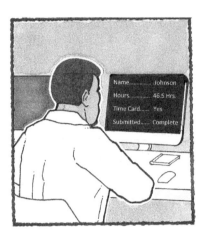

Figure 6.3 "Independent group contingencies are often used in workplaces, on teams, and in classrooms."

  - **Examples:**

    - In order to decrease young individuals using tobacco products, states, with the help of their public health departments, put laws in place stating anyone under 21 may not buy or sell tobacco products.
    - Evan is nervous to start a new job in the city. She is especially concerned about having to possibly parallel park. She watches videos on how to parallel park and practices a few times per week in order to get better. Watching videos and practicing parallel parking are independent variables.

  - **See:** Behavior plan, dependent variable, and intervention

- **Indirect Measurement**

  - **Translation:**

    - Measuring a behavior but not actually watching it happen. You usually get the information from someone else.

  - **Examples:**

    - Sam is a teacher and wants to make sure his students complete their homework. He has them complete a worksheet at home. Sam did not see his students complete the worksheets, but he can see if they are finished or not.
    - You are analyzing eyewitness reports of a crime, but you did not witness the crime yourself.

  - **See:** Data and direct measurement

- **Interdependent Group Contingency**

  - **Translation:**

    - If all members of the group meet the expectations, then they will earn the reward/punisher.

  - **Examples:**

    - A neighborhood pool requires everyone to exit the water during the 10-minute safety break before they can start the break. If everyone is not out of the water within one minute of the whistle blowing, the lifeguards add one minute to the required break time.
    - At restaurants, sometimes they have policies where all members of a party must be present in order to be seated at their table.

  - **See:** Dependent group contingency, group contingency, and independent group contingency

- **Intermittent Reinforcement**

  - **Translations:**

    - Not continuously rewarding a behavior
    - Rewarding behaviors/responses some of the time
    - Variable rewards (Clear, 2018)

  - **Examples:**

    - Scrolling through social media, you're going to come across your favorite videos and pictures once in a while.
    - Jake is working with a client to increase her habit of waking up at 6 am. Jake's behavior analyst has instructed him to send the client five dollars from the reward fund about every two or three days his client wakes up at the correct time.

  - **See:** Continuous reinforcement, reinforcement, and schedules of reinforcement

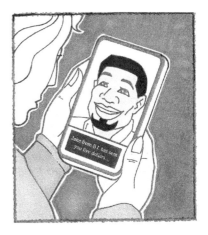

Figure 6.4 "When you're rewarded but you just don't know exactly when you're going to be rewarded keeps you very motivated."

- **Interobserver Agreement (IOA)**

  - **Translation:**

    - A way to measure if two people are taking data the same way

  - **Examples:**

    - A behavior analyst and another therapist took data during a session to see if they were collecting the same information on their client's inappropriate urination behavior.

- Two behavior analysts want to decrease the amount of time people run their water at home. They take data to see if they are collecting the same information on how long people wash their dishes with the water running.

- **See:** Data and treatment integrity/procedural fidelity

- **Interresponse Time (IRT)**

  - **Translation:**

    - The time in between two of the same behaviors/habits

  - **Examples:**

    - Dennis Rader, also known as the blind, torcher, and kill (BTK) serial killer, would wait months or even years in between murdering his next victims (Sederstrom, 2018).
    - A behavior analyst is working with a client who is trying to increase her hydration. The behavior analyst finds it takes her client about five hours between finishing two glasses of water.

  - **See:** Data, duration, frequency, latency, and magnitude

- **Intervention**

  - **Translations:**

    - Curriculum
    - Change plan
    - Lesson plan
    - Performance plan
    - Procedure
    - Remedy
    - Strategy
    - Teaching plan/strategy
    - Treatment

  - **Examples:**

    - Billy is working with the government to decrease child maltreatment. Part of his plan is to create a course for teaching parents how to improve their parent-child interactions, as well as doing randomized in-home checks. These plans would be his intervention.
    - A behavior analyst is working with athletes who are experiencing mental blocks in their sport, also known as the "yips." These mental blocks are causing the athletes to be unable to demonstrate basic skills (e.g., throwing a ball to first base, doing a backbend, putting a golf ball, etc.). The behavior

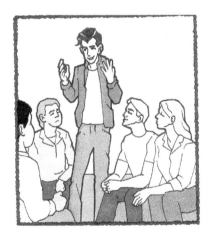

Figure 6.5 "When targeting behavior change, one must implement proactive and reactive strategies."

analyst has put together a plan, or intervention, that includes shaping and reward techniques to help the athletes overcome this issue.

- **See:** Antecedent intervention, behavior plan, proactive, and reactive

- **Intraverbal**

  - **Translations:**

    - Filling in a part of a phrase, line, lyric, etc.
    - Having an exchange with another person

  - **Examples:**

    - Rose is being trained in customer service. Any time a customer calls or emails her with a complaint, her trainer has taught her to say, "I'm sorry to hear that. Let me help you."
    - Taylor Swift is singing at her concert. She sings the lyrics, "It's a cruel.." and the crowd yells back, "SUMMER!" (Swift et al., 2019).

  - **See:** Verbal behavior

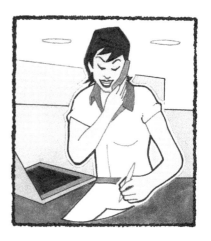

Figure 6.6 "Any back-and-forth exchanges with another person which do not look or sound the same can count as an intraverbal."

References

Al-Nasser, T., Williams, W. L., & Feeney, B. (2019). A brief evaluation of a pictorially enhanced self-instruction packet on participant fidelity across multiple ABA procedures. *Behavior Analysis in Practice, 12*(2), 387–395. https://doi.org/10.1007/s40617-018-00282-w

Bailey, J. S. (1991). Marketing behavior analysis requires different talk. *Journal of Applied Behavior Analysis, 24*(3), 445–448. https://doi.org/10.1901/jaba.1991.24-445

Clear, J. (2018). *Atomic habits: An easy and proven way to build good habits and break bad ones.* Avery, an imprint of Penguin Random House.

Fowler, S. A. (1991). Behavior analysis in education and public policy: A necessary intersection. In R. Gardner, III, D. M. Sainato, J. O. Cooper, T. E. Heron, W. L. Heward, J. W. Eshleman, & T. A. Grossi (Eds.), *Behavior analysis in education* (pp. 367–372). Books/Cole.

Foxx, R. M. (1996). Translating the covenant: The behavior analyst as ambassador and translator. *The Behavior Analyst, 19*(2), 147–161. https://doi.org/10.1007/BF03393162

Graff, R. B., & Karsten, A. M. (2012). Evaluation of a self-instruction package for conducting stimulus preference assessments. *Journal of Applied Behavior Analysis, 45*(1), 69–82. https://doi.org/10.1901/jaba.2012.45-69

Lerman, D. C. (2023). Putting the power of behavior analysis in the hands of nonbehavioral professionals: Toward a blueprint for dissemination. *Journal of Applied Behavior Analysis, 57*(1), 1–16. https://doi.org/10.1002/jaba.1036

Lindsley, O. R. (1991). From technical jargon to plain English for application. *Journal of Applied Behavior Analysis, 24*(3), 449–458. https://doi.org/10.1901/jaba.1991.24-449

Marshall, K. B. (2021). *The impact of behavior analysis jargon on the effective training of stakeholders* [Doctoral dissertation, Endicott College]. ProQuest. https://www.proquest.com/docview/2571066257?pq-origsite=gscholar&fromopenview=true

Sederstrom, J. (2018). *Why did Dennis Rader, the BTK killer, wait so long in between his murders?* https://www.oxygen.com/martinis-murder/dennis-rader-btk-killer-wait-so-long-between-his-murder-victims

Smith, J. M. (2016). Strategies to position behavior analysis as the contemporary science of what works in behavior change. *The Behavior Analyst*, *39*(1), 75–87. https://doi.org/10.1007/s40614-015-0044-3

Swift, T., Antonoff, J. M., & Clark, A. (2019). Cruel Summer [Recorded by T. Swift, J. M. Antonoff, A. Clark & M. Riddleberger]. On *Lover* [Medium of recording]. Republic Records.

7   Please, Thank You, and No Fancy Words

Behavior analysts, just like any other professionals, need to exhibit appropriate, professional etiquette (i.e., the way in which we behave in a professional or business setting) (Bailey & Burch, 2023). Experts have said that in order to uphold the highest level of professional etiquette, one of the behaviors we should demonstrate is communicating well, without jargon (Bailey & Burch, 2023). In recent findings, researchers concluded that using behavior analytic jargon can be hard to understand and off-putting to the general public (Friman, 2006, 2021; Marshall, 2021). It can also imply inaccurate values of science and decrease the acceptability of behavior analytic services (Becirevic et al., 2016; Marshall, 2021). For example, people may think we simply want to control others, change people's personalities, or assume we don't take individual needs into consideration when creating curriculum. I have heard all of these comments in many conversations throughout my career and have seen social media posts with these same notes. "What makes a good behavior analyst can be bad for public relations" (Foxx, 1996, p. 149).

Dr. Jon Bailey, an expert behavior analyst and leader in the field, attended an animal performance at Cypress Gardens and witnessed the trainers changing the term "operant conditioning" to "affection training" (Bailey, 1991). When he asked the trainer after the performance why she didn't use "operant conditioning" to explain how she trained the birds, she said, "We don't want to confuse the audience and complicate matters" (Bailey, 1991, p. 445). Operant conditioning is only a familiar term to a relative few. Many people have used operant conditioning in their lives (e.g., onboarding a new hire and teaching someone how to do a cartwheel) but would refer to it as "coaching," "training," or something similar to make it easily understood for their audience. If nonbehavior analysts who use the science and are changing the terminology, this is an obvious sign that we need to start speaking differently.

Terms and Translations

- **Latency**
  - **Translation:**
    - The time in between a cue, prompt, request, or demand and the person responding
  - **Examples:**
    - The five seconds between the time I text my mom and when she responds to me is the latency.

DOI: 10.4324/9781003439776-7

- The time in between when the World Health Organization (WHO) declares there is a new pandemic and what to do to stay safe and the countries of the world putting safety procedures in place is the latency. Sometimes, the response time is quick, other times it is more delayed.

- **See:** Data and direct measurement

- **Magnitude**

  - **Translation:**

    - Measuring the amount of intensity or force of an action/behavior

  - **Examples:**

    - When you go to a professional sports game, the team may have a "scream meter," which will measure how loud the crowd is screaming.
    - Hunter, a toddler, may push down harder with his crayons on paper compared to his father, Anthony, who knows you don't have to apply much pressure to the paper in order to color a picture.

  - **See:** Data and direct measurement

- **Maintenance**

  - **Translation:**

    - Once the teaching portion has stopped, the learner is able to demonstrate this skill/ behavior without needing help.

  - **Examples:**

    - BCBAs were trained on the new scheduling system. One month later, when supervisors checked on them, they were still using the system correctly.
    - Billy taught a client how to engage in coping skills to help with social anxiety when in large crowds. Billy ends up going to a crowded concert venue a few months later with his client and notices he is taking deep breaths and calming down on his own. Yes!

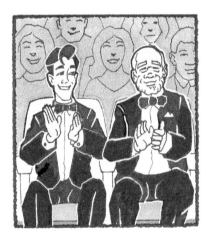

Figure 7.1 "Being able to maintain a skill and demonstrate it independently is one of the ultimate goals of behavior change."

  - **See:** Baseline, generalization, and intervention

- **Mand**

  - **Translation:**

    - Asking or telling someone what you need/want

  - **Examples:**

    - I attended a Cinco de Mayo party in college. The police and campus security showed up, so some of my friends lifted the garage door and yelled, "¡Vámanos!"

which in Spanish means, "Let's go!" My friends manded for all of us to go and run from the house.

- The Hawaiian environmental workers made an announcement stating, "Anyone going to the beaches or swimming in the ocean needs to use reef safe sunscreen." The workers manded that the public use a specific kind of sunscreen to protect the ocean's reef from bleaching.

- **See:** Functional communication training and verbal behavior

- **Momentary Time Sampling**

  - **Translation:**

    - Tracking if a specific behavior/habit happened at the very beginning or end of a block of time

  - **Examples:**

    - Coach Mike has a timer set for five minutes. He is trying to track if one of his players has her eyes on the game instead of the crowd. Once the five minutes are up, he immediately looks up to see if his player is paying attention to the game or to the crowd. She was talking to a fan in the stands. Classic.
    - A behavior analyst in a nursing home is working with a few clients who have been taking items out of other people's rooms without asking. She sits in the hallway by all of the rooms and sets a timer for three minutes. When the timer goes off, she checks all of the rooms in the hall to see if anyone is in a room they shouldn't be.

  - **See:** Discontinuous measurement, partial-interval recording, and whole interval recording

- **Motivating Operation (MO)**

  - **Translations:**

    - A craving (Clear, 2018)
    - A motive
    - An aspect of the environment that determines how often a particular behavior occurs and how valuable a reward is
    - The motivation behind doing anything

  - **Examples:**

    - When she's tired, Carson is more likely to do less work. Taking breaks will be extremely motivating to her and will probably happen more frequently during this time.
    - Getting into a speakeasy club makes getting the password extremely motivating. I'm also more likely to go back to the club when I am in the mood to dance.

  - **See:** Abolishing operation, conditioned motivating operation, establishing operation,

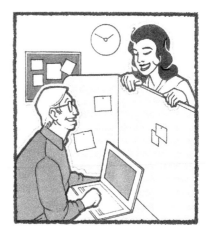

Figure 7.2 "Taking breaks is good, but when you're tired, taking breaks is even more motivating especially when your friends are close by."

reflexive conditioned motivating operation, transitive conditioned motivating operation, and unconditioned motivating operation

- **Negative Punishment**

  - **Translations:**

    - Fine
    - Penalty
    - Removing desirable things to get someone to stop behaving a certain way.
    - Taking away something someone likes to make it less likely that they will do a particular behavior again.

  - **Examples:**

    - A brother and sister are yelling at each other over who gets to watch the iPad. Their dad takes the iPad away to get the yelling to stop. The brother and sister are less likely to yell at each other over the iPad in the future.
    - Carson's company takes PTO time from employees for coming into work late in hopes this will stop employees from showing up late.

  - **See:** Positive punishment, punishment, response blocking, and response cost

- **Negative Reinforcement**

  - **Translations:**

    - A solution to a problem
    - Getting relief from or avoiding something you do not like (e.g., person, place, and feeling), which makes you more likely to respond this way again.
    - Relief

  - **Examples:**

    - Emily puts headphones on in the car to drown out the sound of her kids yelling at each other in the backseat. She is able to relax while she is driving now. Emily is more likely to put her headphones on the next time her kids yell at each other to get relief from the loud arguing and to help her relax.
    - The softball team Carson helps does not like to do their daily mile run at the end

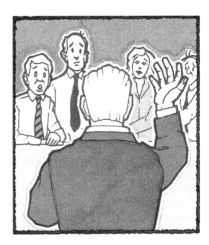

Figure 7.3 "Sometimes incentives are taken away, which can be an example of negative punishment."

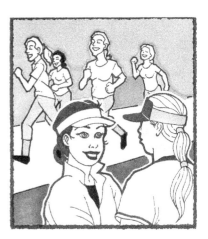

Figure 7.4 "Adding incentives to a team's practice plan can help them stay on track to meet their goals and keep them motivated."

of practice. If the team makes three or less mistakes in practice, she has instructed their coach to only have the girls run half a mile. Removing it in the long run will likely increase the team's motivation to make all of their plays in practice.

- **See:** Noncontingent reinforcement, positive reinforcement, and reinforcement

- **Noncontingent Reinforcement (NCR)**
  - **Translations:**
    - Rewards given to you on a schedule regardless of the behavior you are engaged in
    - Distractors
  - **Examples:**

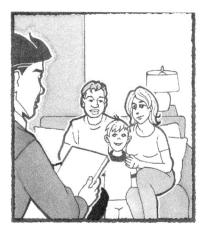

- Billy is working with his four-year-old client, who has limited communication skills. The client screams in order to gain others' attention about every seven minutes. Billy instructs the family to give their child attention (i.e., hugs, kisses, and talking to him) about every five minutes. Once the family reports that their child is no longer screaming, Billy directs the family to give their child attention less often.
- A behavior technician is working with a student who threatens his classmates to get out of having to do his school work (about every ten minutes). The BCBA has instructed the technician to allow the student to take a break from his work about every seven minutes.

Figure 7.5 "Scheduled incentives can help decrease someone's motivation for engaging in challenging behaviors, such as screaming."

- **See:** Antecedent interventions and reinforcement

References

Bailey, J. S. (1991). Marketing behavior analysis requires different talk. *Journal of Applied Behavior Analysis, 24*(3), 445–448. https://doi.org/10.1901/jaba.1991.24-445

Bailey, J. S., & Burch, M. R. (2023). *25 essential skills for the successful behavior analyst: From graduate school to chief executive officer* (2nd ed.). Routledge.

Becirevic, A., Critchfield, T. S., & Reed, D. D. (2016). On the social acceptability of behavior analytic terms: Crowdsourced comparisons of lay and technical language. *The Behavior Analyst, 39*(2), 305–317. https://doi.org/10.1007/s40614-016-0067-4

Clear, J. (2018) *Atomic habits: An easy and proven way to build good habits and break bad ones.* Avery, an imprint of Penguin Random House.

Foxx, R. M. (1996). Translating the covenant: The behavior analyst as ambassador and translator. *The Behavior Analyst, 19*(2), 147–161. https://doi.org/10.1007/BF03393162

Friman, P. C. (2006). Eschew obfuscation: A colloquial description of contingent reinforcement. *European Journal of Behavior Analysis, 7*(2), 107–109.

Friman, P. C. (2021). There is no such thing as a bad boy: The circumstances view of problem behavior. *Journal of Applied Behavior Analysis*, *54*(2), 636–653. https://doi.org/10.1002/jaba.816

Marshall, K. B. (2021). *The impact of behavior analysis jargon on the effective training of stakeholders* [Doctoral dissertation, Endicott College]. ProQuest. https://www.proquest.com/docview/2571066257?pq-origsite=gscholar&fromopenview=true

8 Different Definitions

Have you ever heard someone use the word "reinforcement" in a sentence, but they actually meant to say "punishment?" For example, "My class was misbehaving so much today that I had to reinforce them to make it stop." Playing and coaching softball for years, I've come across many coaches who have said things like, "We're going to have to use some reinforcement, like running, to make sure these mistakes don't happen again." They really meant to say "punishment." I've witnessed this countless times in professional and social settings. It is a perfect example of how the general public interprets the meaning of certain behavior analytic terms differently compared to individuals who work in the field (Marshall, 2021). Additionally, behavior analysts have taken words from other professions and changed their meanings to them to align with our science. For instance, one of the definitions of "extinction" from dictionary.com states, "the process of becoming extinct; a coming to an end or dying out of a species" (2020). The definition of extinction behavior analysts use is "The discontinuing of reinforcement for a previously reinforced behavior" (Cooper et al., 2007, p. 695). This can lead to confusion and other negative effects when scientists attempt to disseminate behavior analysis information (Marshall, 2021).

Fewer problems occur when new terms or labels are created instead of changing the meaning of existing words (Deitz & Arrington, 1983; Foxx, 1996). Foxx (1996) suggested we create retronyms for our behavior analysis terminology. Retronyms are words that are created to fit the times or new terms to describe old ones (Foxx, 1996). Also, misunderstanding these terms has the potential to harm the connections between behavior analysts and others (Marshall, 2021). "It is reasonable to suggest that productive collaboration requires conversation, a core prerequisite of which would seem to be reliance on mutually acceptable and understandable terms" (Becirevic et al., 2016, p. 312). Currently, there are many behavior analysts who are working tirelessly to grow the field. The last thing we want is to confuse people about our science. Using language that everyone can understand will help behavior analysts avoid these setbacks and potentially expand the field even more.

Terms and Translations

- **Observer Drift**
  - **Translation:**
    - A change in the way someone is tracking a behavior different from how they were trained, which is usually an error

DOI: 10.4324/9781003439776-8

- **Examples:**
  - If I was measuring how often my husband played video games, I would take data on when he plays games on his PlayStation and on his phone. If I started to forget to track him playing games on his phone, this would be observer drift.
  - Brent is partnering with environmental workers to clean the ocean of plastics and other pollutants. He coaches his assistant how to track the types of pollutants they are collecting each day. Brent's assistant starts taking data on only glass bottles instead of plastic, glass, and tin bottles or cans. The change in data collection is observer drift.
- **See:** Data, direct measurement, and indirect measurement

- **Operant Conditioning**
  - **Translations:**
    - Learning by consequences, such as rewards or punishers
    - When the consequences of a behavior/habit either increase or decrease the likelihood of it happening again
    - When the consequences make it more or less likely for you to behave a certain way again
  - **Examples:**
    - Brian has learned he will willingly work longer hours when he is paid hourly or by commission compared to if he is a salaried worker.
    - Dale is less likely to swim at her friend's pool because the last time she was there, many strands of hair were found in the pool. Wet hair grosses Dale out.
  - **See:** Classical conditioning, consequence, reinforcement, and punishment

- **Overcorrection**
  - **Translation:**
    - Redoing a behavior, a certain number of times, in order to make an inappropriate behavior less likely to happen again in the future.
  - **Examples:**
    - In the movie *Madeline,* Madeline and her classmates get in trouble for breaking the rules of the school, so their teacher has them write, "I will follow the school rules and will never do (name of problem behavior) again," about 50 times.
    - A doctor's assistant forgets to call in a prescription for a patient. The doctor has her assistant practice calling the pharmacy immediately after the doctor has finished the prescription three times before finishing the rest of her work.
  - **See:** Positive punishment, punishment, and restitution overcorrection

- **Parsimony**
  - **Translations:**
    - Ruling out the simplest explanations and strategies before considering more complex options
    - The simplest explanation should be considered first.

- **Examples:**

  - Jessica was working with a client who was touching his genitals in public. A lot of the therapists thought it was possible masturbation and other more complicated reasons for occurring. Jessica suggested he might just be itchy or have to go to the bathroom. He did indeed have to go to the bathroom, so she taught him how to access the bathroom on his own.
  - People spot a celebrity on the red carpet twirling in her dress and laughing extremely loud. The simplest explanation as to why this celebrity is twirling and laughing loudly is to gain attention from the photographers and other people watching.

- **Partial-Interval Recording**

  - **Translation:**

    - The recorder will mark if a behavior happened but not specifically how many times it happened during short blocks of time.

  - **Examples:**

    - Carrie is working with a client who has a tendency to say "um" and "like" often when he speaks to other people. She wants to take initial data to track these behaviors. She set small periods of time during their sessions to track if her client said these words in his sentences. If her client did say "um" or "like," Carrie would mark this on her data sheet.
    - Gwen is working with an entire floor of clients who have traumatic brain injuries. Her clients often start tasks and walk away from them. Gwen sets small blocks of time during their independent work tasks and marks if they remain on task for any period of time.

  - **See:** Discontinuous measurement, momentary time sampling, and whole interval recording

- **Pivotal Behavior**

  - **Translations:**

    - A behavior or skill you were taught that leads you to try other, similar behaviors/ skills on your own
    - A new version of what you were originally taught to do
    - When you learn one skill and start to do different variations of that skill on your own

  - **Examples:**

    - You were taught how to sing a few basic pop songs. You loved singing so much that you started trying other genres of music to sing to, such as opera, country, and hip-hop.

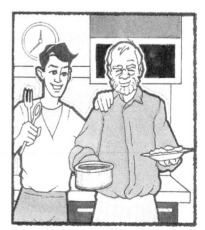

Figure 8.1 "Trying new recipes after being taught a couple of basic ones is a perfect example of pivotal behavior."

- Billy teaches his client how to make simple sandwich and breakfast recipes. The client has also tried to make himself pasta and soup recipes without the help from Billy.

- **See:** Behavioral cusp and response generalization

- **Planned Ignoring**

  - **Translation:**

    - When attention or physical interaction is scheduled to be paused until an undesired behavior stops

  - **Examples:**

    - Researchers conducted a study with an individual who had schizophrenia and engaged in bizarre vocalizations (Wilder et al., 2013). They found that his unusual comments were maintained by other people's attention, and one of the ways they worked to decrease his bizarre vocalizations was to not respond to them, also known as planned ignoring (Wilder et al., 2001).
    - When I pitched in games, there were many opponents I played against and fans who would scream mean things at me. I would deliberately not look at them or respond back to them. I would just strike everyone out and move onto the next hitter. Boom, roasted.

  - **See:** Negative punishment, punishment, and response cost

- **Positive Punishment**

  - **Translations:**

    - Adding something unpleasant to make it less likely that a behavior will happen again in the future
    - Decreasing the likelihood of a behavior happening again by adding something you don't like to the situation

  - **Examples:**

    - A teacher giving a student extra homework when they forgot to do the original assignment. This will hopefully make it less likely that the student will forget to do their homework again.
    - At Billy's workplace, staff members have to stay late to clean the office kitchen if they left their garbage there during the week to make it less likely they will make a mess again.

  - **See:** Negative punishment, overcorrection, punishment, response blocking, and restitution overcorrection

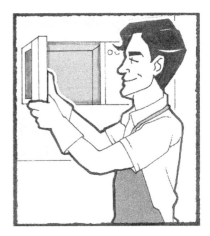

Figure 8.2 "Having to clean the office microwave, when it is rarely ever cleaned, can be a very tedious task. A task that not many people would want to do after working a long day."

- **Positive Reinforcement**

  - **Translations:**

    - Adding something desirable to make it more likely that a behavior will happen again in the future
    - Increasing the likelihood of a behavior happening by adding something you like to the situation

  - **Examples:**

    - PJ gets weekly massages and they feel amazing. She is more likely to go back to the same massage therapist because she had such a great experience.
    - Gaining followers on social media for posting videos about behavior science will make it more likely for me to post more videos on the same topic.

  - **See:** Access-maintained behaviors, behavior, differential reinforcement, negative reinforcement, noncontingent reinforcement, and reinforcement

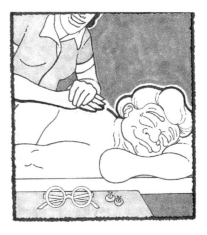

Figure 8.3 "The more you enjoy something, or gain reinforcement, the more you want to do it again and again."

- **Premack Principle**

  - **Translations:**

    - First do X, then you get Y.
    - Doing a less preferred activity, followed by a highly preferred activity; over time, this increases the less preferred activity and can lead to it becoming fun or desired.
    - Linking a behavior you want to do with one you need to do in order to make the one you need to do more desirable over time (Clear, 2018)
    - Temptation bundling (Clear, 2018)

  - **Examples:**

    - Jackie's grandchildren are very messy when they visit, they leave toys all over the house and do not keep their rooms neat, so she has a new rule "No eating Grandma's cookies (a highly preferred activity) until everything is put away (a less preferred activity). Her grandchildren have started to keep the house very clean when they come over and now don't mind cleaning up. Go Gramcracker!
    - Shelby didn't like to exercise (a less preferred activity), so she set up a system where if she worked out four out of five days, she could go dancing with her friends on the weekend (a highly preferred activity).

  - **See:** Behavior, contingency, establishing operation, and reinforcement

- **Private Events**
  - **Translation:**
    - Thoughts and feelings other people cannot see inside of you or another person
  - **Examples:**
    - Jake having positive or negative thoughts
    - Feeling pleasure from having sex
  - **See:** Behavior
- **Proactive**
  - **Translation:**
    - Preventing issues before they occur
  - **Examples:**
    - Putting deodorant on <u>before</u> you exercise to prevent body odor.
    - Researchers suggest removing lethal items from the home to prevent suicide as well as harm to others, such as guns, medications, and alcohol (Rynyan et al., 2017).
  - **See:** Negative reinforcement and reactive

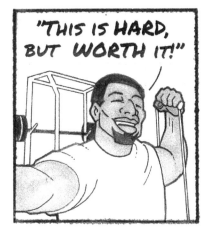

Figure 8.4 "Many thoughts can go through your head when you're working out, such as "It's really hot in here" or "I'm going to look great for bikini season," which are examples of private events."

- **Program**
  - **Translation:**
    - A written plan to teach one specific behavior, habit, or skill, which usually includes:
      - Materials required and how to arrange them
      - How to cue or prompt a response to happen
      - Identify the response you are targeting
      - Describe how to reward the correct response
      - Describe how to correct errors when they occur
  - **Examples:**
    - Kim is a BCBA who is teaching Adam how to wait for another person's attention. She writes a ten-step plan or program to teach Adam how to apply this skill with others in his life.
    - A therapist has a client who does not like to leave his house. The therapist writes a plan to have his client open the door, then step on to the porch, then walk to the mailbox, and finally leave the house and walk to a neighbor's house down the street at least once per day. Over time, the therapist increases the criteria in the program for his client to travel further and for longer periods of time to help his client become more comfortable with leaving the house to visit his friends and go shopping.
  - **See:** Behavior, behavior skills training, error correction, intervention, and prompt

- **Prompt**
  - **Translations:**
    - Cue
    - Direction
    - Reminder
    - Signal
  - **Examples:**
    - Setting an alarm to remind myself to text my sister
    - Planned Parenthood posting a billboard reminding people to come to their facilities to get testing for sexually transmitted diseases and treatment

- **Punishment**
  - **Translations:**
    - A strategy to decrease actions or behaviors
    - Correction
  - **Examples:**
    - The police department giving speeding tickets to drivers for driving too fast in order to get drivers to slow down in the future
    - Sarah losing the privilege of driving her car this weekend since she was late for curfew last weekend
  - **See:** Negative punishment, overcorrection, planned ignoring, positive punishment, response cost, response blocking, and restitution overcorrection

- **Punisher**
  - **Translations:**
    - Demerit
    - Deterrent
    - Discourager
    - Fine
    - Penalty
    - Repercussion
    - Sanction
  - **Examples:**
    - Being removed from a sporting event for running on the field
    - Receiving an after-school detention for cheating on a test
  - **See:** Punishment

References

Becirevic, A., Critchfield, T. S., & Reed, D. D. (2016). On the social acceptability of behavior analytic terms: Crowdsourced comparisons of lay and technical language. *The Behavior Analyst*, *39*(2), 305–317. https://doi.org/10.1007/s40614-016-0067-4

Clear, J. (2018) *Atomic habits: An easy and proven way to build good habits and break bad ones.* Avery, an imprint of Penguin Random House.

Cooper, J. O., Heron, T. E., & Heward, W. L. (eds.). (2007). *Applied behavior analysis* (2nd ed.). Merrill Prentice Hall.

Deitz, S. M., & Arrington, R. L. (1983). Factors confusing language use in analysis of behavior. *Behaviorism, 11*(2), 117–132.

Extinction. (2020). In *Dictionary.com.* Retrieved January 30, 2024, from https://www.dictionary.com/browse/extinction

Foxx, R. M. (1996). Translating the covenant: The behavior analyst as ambassador and translator. *The Behavior Analyst, 19*(2), 147–161. https://doi.org/10.1007/BF03393162

Marshall, K. B. (2021). *The impact of behavior analysis jargon on the effective training of stakeholders* [Doctoral dissertation, Endicott College]. ProQuest. https://www.proquest.com/docview/2571066257?pq-origsite=gscholar&fromopenview=true

Rynyan, C. W., Brooks-Russell, A., & Brandspigel, S. (2017). Law enforcement and gun retailers as partners for safely storing guns to prevent suicide: A study in 8 mountain West States. *American Journal of Public Health, 107*(11), 1789–1794. https://apha.org/-/media/Files/PDF/topics/Suicide_Prevention.ashx

Wilder, D. A., Masuda, A., O'Connor, C., & Baham, M. (2013). Brief functional analysis and treatment of bizarre vocalizations in an adult with schizophrenia. *Journal of Applied Behavior Analysis, 34*(1), 65–68. https://doi.org/10.1901/jaba.2001.34-65

9 Is There a Word for That?

Behavior analytic jargon can be challenging to understand, even for someone with a vast psychology background. To make matters even more difficult, try to translate behavior analytic jargon into another language. It is a nearly impossible task. I've heard from my friends and others around me who learned English as a second language that English is one of the most challenging languages to master. This is partly due to the multiple definitions for a single word. As previously stated, behavior analysis is guilty of adopting already existing words and changing the definitions to fit our science, making matters even more difficult for those who are attempting to master the English language.

Many of my past bilingual clients had difficulty trying to grasp the concept of behavior analysis while also attempting to understand the treatments myself and my colleagues were suggesting. I'm sure this was partly due to the confusing ABA terminology that was used. What helped me immensely in these situations was using language from this book to explain behavior analysis basically and the plans I developed. Using visuals to support the information was a huge aid too. Additionally, I've had co-workers in the past who stepped in as translators for our clients who were not fluent in English. They asked me so many times if there were translational resources to help them speak with our clients more easily. I wish I had this book to give them at the time because it would have been so helpful. Although I can't go back in time and hand my co-workers this book, I know it will greatly aid them in their next conversations with their clients and hope it helps you too!

Terms and Translations

- **Rate**
  - **Translation:**
    - How often a behavior happens in a specific time period
  - **Examples:**
    - My favorite podcast, *Small Town Murder*, posts a new episode once per week. The rate of podcast posts for this show is once per week.
    - A school receives reports from teachers that there are many occurrences of bullying happening. A behavior analyst takes data and finds there are on average five bullying incidents per day.
  - **See:** Behavior, data, direct measurement, and frequency

DOI: 10.4324/9781003439776-9

- **Reactive**
  - **Translations:**
    - Reacting
    - Responding after a behavior
  - **Examples:**
    - Dawn is addicted to cigarettes. She recently joined a program to help her stop smoking. At Dawn's check-ins, after she produces a negative drug test, she is rewarded with cash or gift cards. The reaction after Dawn tested negative was rewarding for her.
    - After you vote at your local polling location, you are given a sticker that says, "I voted!"
  - **See:** Behavior, consequence, and proactive

- **Reactivity**
  - **Translation:**
    - Acting or behaving differently because people are watching you
  - **Examples:**
    - People often act differently when posting on social media, such as by only sharing the good parts of their day in their videos or using aggressive/accusatory language when commenting on others' posts. This differs from when they are talking with their family or close friends.
    - Employees may socialize less when their boss is present compared to when he is not.
  - **See:** Behavior

- **Reflexive Conditioned Motivating Operation**
  - **Translations:**
    - A warning signal that a situation is going to get better or worse. This can affect what you are motivated to do next.
    - Red or white flag
  - **Examples:**
    - When the COVID-19 pandemic was announced, which was a warning sign, people rushed to the grocery stores and bought excess amounts of toilet paper and cleaning supplies.
    - Jake knows if he doesn't get to the bar by 9 pm, they will charge him a cover fee. He makes sure to get ready quickly and arrive at the bar before 9 pm so he doesn't have to pay the bouncer $20.

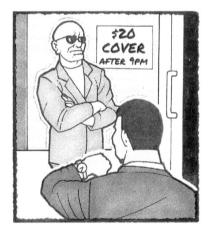

Figure 9.1 "No one wants to pay a cover, which is why many people either try to get to the bar early or choose bars that don't have an extra fee to enter."

- **See:** Conditioned motivating operation, motivating operation, and transitive motivating operation

- **Registered Behavior Technician**

  - **Translation:**

    - An individual who administers or implements behavioral strategies/treatments made by a behavior analyst

  - **Examples:**

    - In hospital and medical settings, a doctor will recommend a specific treatment for a patient and the nurses will administer the treatment. Behavior technicians are the nurses of the behavior analysis field. They administer behavioral treatments to clients under the supervision of a behavior analyst but do not create treatment plans.
    - Bob is a behavior technician who works with his BCBA, Jude. Jude has created a behavior plan for a client experiencing behavioral issues from his depression. Bob goes to the client's house to implement the behavior treatment Jude created.

  - **See:** Board-certified assistance behavior analyst and board-certified behavior analyst

- **Reinforcement**

  - **Translations:**

    - A strategy to increase behavior
    - Encouragement
    - Gratification
    - Incentivizing
    - Reward
    - Satisfaction

  - **Examples:**

    - A professor awards extra credit to her students for participating in her research project.
    - Dale does not like to hold cold drinks. Her mom tells Dale that if she puts a paper towel around the glass, her hands won't become as cold. Dale tries this out and is now more likely to use a paper towel in the future when holding a drink to avoid her hands becoming cold.

  - **See:** Behavior, differential reinforcement, negative reinforcement, non-contingent reinforcement, and positive reinforcement

- **Reinforcer**

  - **Translations:**

    - Encouragement
    - Incentive
    - Motivator
    - Reward
    - What is being used to increase the likelihood of a behavior/habit to happen again

- **Examples:**

  - Will gives his new puppy, Payton, treats every few steps she stays next to him on their walk. This is done to make it more likely that Payton stays next to Will when they walk together. The treats are Payton's reinforcer for walking next to Will.
  - Lindsay wants to wake up earlier in the morning. Every time she wakes up before 6 am, she grabs her favorite book and starts to read. Reading her favorite book is Lindsay's reinforcer for waking up at her goal time.

- **See:** Reinforcement

- **Repertoire:**

  - **Translation:**

    - All behaviors or skills a person can perform

  - **Examples:**

    - Skills some 1st graders can perform include:

      - Counting to 100
      - Subtracting numbers
      - Naming different coins
      - Naming the colors of the rainbow
      - Lining up with their class to go to recess

    - Some skills Jake, a behavior technician, should be able to perform include:

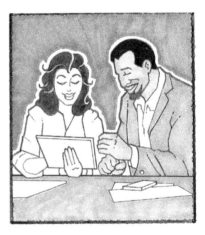

      - Reading and implementing a treatment plan
      - Taking data
      - Writing a summary of their sessions
      - Debriefing clients on their progress after sessions
      - Asking their supervisor for help

  - **See:** Behavior

Figure 9.2 "Registered behavior technicians often collaborate with their supervising behavior analysts to ensure they are implementing treatment plans and collecting data correctly."

- **Respondent Behavior**

  - **Translations:**

    - An automatic response to something you've sensed
    - A reflex

  - **Examples:**

    - Blinking when your eyes are dry
    - Yawning when you are tired

  - **See:** Behavior, classical conditioning, and response

- **Response Blocking**
  - **Translation:**
    - Physically blocking or stopping a behavior
  - **Examples:**
    - The security guard putting their arm in front of me so I don't get any closer to the stage during a concert.
    - A child tries to put beads in her nose, so her mother puts her hand in front of the child's face.
  - **See:** Negative punishment, positive punishment, and punishment
- **Response Class**
  - **Translation:**
    - Behaviors that look different but happen for the same reason
  - **Examples:**
    - I can do yoga or lift weights in order to stay in shape.
    - PJ puts on sunscreen or sits in the shade in order to avoid sunburn.
  - **See:** Behavior, function, functionally equivalent/ compatible, and reinforcement

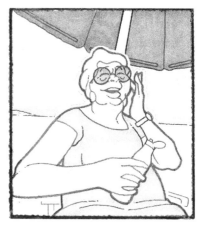

Figure 9.3 "We do certain things for the same reason or to get the same result, such as sitting in the shade and wearing sunscreen to avoid sun damage on our skin."

- **Response Cost**
  - **Translations:**
    - Taking away something preferred due to an undesirable behavior/habit happening
    - A fine
  - **Examples:**
    - Paying a cancellation fee for missing your doctor's appointment
    - Not being allowed back to your favorite bar because you "acted up" the last time you partied there
  - **See:** Negative punishment, planned ignoring, positive punishment, and punishment
- **Response Generalization**
  - **Translation:**
    - A new version of what you were originally taught to do
    - Performing different variations of a behavior/habit

- **Examples:**

  - In driving school, you were taught to hold the steering wheel with both hands on the sides of the wheel. After passing the driving exam, you sometimes hold your hands in at the bottom or even the top of the steering wheel.
  - In the past, students were taught to look up information using encyclopedias, Google or other search engines. Now, the same people use other resources to find information, such as social media and artificial intelligence.

- **See:** Generalization, pivotal behavior, stimulus generalization, and stimulus

- **Restitution Overcorrection**[1]

  - **Translation:**

    - Repairing damage or making the environment better than it was before an undesired behavior occurred

  - **Examples:**

    - Andy punched a hole in the wall when he became extremely escalated during an office party. If restitution was used, he would not only have to repair the hole in the wall but he might also have to then paint all of the walls and sanitize everyone's desks too.
    - During homecoming week at my high school, the seniors painted the security hut outside of the school red. The school caught the students and not only made them paint the hut white again, but they also had to paint all of the underground track walls and clean the floors.

  - **See:** Behavior, overcorrection, positive punishment, punishment, and target Behavior

- **Rule Governed Behavior**

  - **Translations:**

    - Acting a certain way because rules or laws are in place, even though you've never been rewarded or punished for following or not following that rule
    - Behavior controlled by rules or laws

  - **Examples:**

    - When you are beginning to learn how to cook, you usually follow recipes exactly. When you become a more seasoned chef, no pun intended, you will rarely use a cook book or recipes and just cook to taste.
    - You see a sign outside of a park that says, "No Trespassing." You've never gone inside the park because of this sign.

  - **See:** Behavior, punishment, and reinforcement

Note

1 This procedure is not recommended. Understanding the reason why a behavior is occurring should be done first before implementing any behavior change strategies.

10   The Other Side of the Argument

The topic of using layman's terms versus technical language has been heavily debated in applied behavior analysis (Bailey, 1991; Branch & Vollmer, 2004; Critchfield, 2014; Friman, 2004; Hayes, 1991; Hineline, 1980; Lindsley, 1991; Marshall, 2021; Risley, 1975). Although there is great importance in being able to speak in layman's terms, some practitioners argue that speaking basically when disseminating behavior science can have negative effects. Some researchers have stated the usage of basic language can decrease the precision of replicating and testing behavior analytic findings (Branch & Vollmer, 2004; Hineline, 1980; Marshall, 2021; Schlinger et al., 1991). For instance, when practitioners create instructions for others to follow, if basic terms are used, others could interpret them differently, which could result in less accurate data collection, treatments may not be as effective, etc. These are all possibilities, but there are ways to bypass these potential issues. First, if consistent language is used when translating jargon, this has the potential to increase accurate usage of behavior analytic strategies and plans. Next, even if consistent jargon is used, there is no guarantee everyone is going to understand it, resulting in more issues. Last, like I mentioned previously, behavior analysts are not the only ones who are implementing their plans. Other people involved in the behavior change process (e.g., teachers, coaches, parents, and department leaders) are the ones taking the plans and using them. If these people do not understand what the directions are telling them to do, there is no point in having a plan at all. If we cannot disseminate our science effectively, there is little reason to keep discovering (Foxx, 1996).

Terms and Translations

- **Satiation**
  - **Translation:**
    - Being overloaded with rewards, making them less desirable
  - **Examples:**
    - You drank a few too many margaritas on Friday after work. You won't want to drink many cocktails on Saturday at brunch because you drank so much the night before.
    - Mike plays fetch a lot with his puppy in the morning. The puppy is tired and does not desire to play fetch in the afternoon because he played so much earlier.
  - **See:** Abolishing operation, behavior, and motivating operation

DOI: 10.4324/9781003439776-10

- **Schedule of Reinforcement**
  - **Translation:**
    - A description of how and when a behavior/habit will be rewarded
  - **Examples:**
    - Receiving commission on every sale you make
    - Receiving pain medication every two hours while you are in the hospital after your surgery
  - **See:** Fixed interval schedule of reinforcement, fixed ratio schedule of reinforcement, variable interval schedule of reinforcement, and variable ratio schedule of reinforcement

- **Self-Management**
  - **Translation:**
    - You managing and changing your own behavior
    - Self-monitoring

  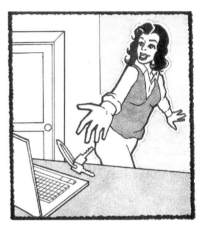

  Figure 10.1 "You can't leave the house without your keys, and you really don't want to leave for work without your laptop. This is a perfect self-management strategy for this kind of situation."

  - **Examples:**
    - Carson puts her keys on top of her laptop to make sure she brings it with her when she leaves for work.
    - Making a to-do list for the week and rewarding myself for finishing everything by going to the mall. Shopping day!
  - **See:** Behavior, behavior plan, habit reversal, and intervention

- **Shaping**
  - **Translation:**
    - Rewarding small steps to teach a larger/more complicated skill
  - **Examples:**
    - Ariana's partner does not put his dirty clothes in the laundry bin, he just leaves them on the floor. Ariana moved the bin to be right next to where he leaves his clothes. He started putting his clothes in the bin. Every so often, Ariana would move the bin closer to the laundry room until the bin was in the laundry room and her partner was consistently putting his dirty clothes in there.

  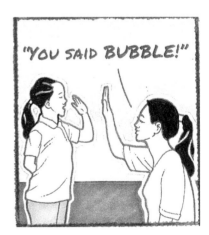

  Figure 10.2 "Taking small steps of progress is one of the best ways to achieve your goals."

- When Rose was little, her mother taught her how to say "bubble" with these steps:

  - Giving Rose a high five after she says, "buh."
  - Giving Rose a high five after she says, "buh-b."
  - Giving Rose a high five after she says, "bubble."

- **See:** Behavior, chaining, and reinforcement

- **Social Significance**

  - **Translations:**

    - Impactful
    - Making an impactful difference
    - Making a meaningful difference
    - Personally meaningful
    - Personally significant
    - When changing a behavior/habit makes a meaningful impact in a person's life

  - **Examples:**

    - Teaching an individual who was not previously able to speak to advocate for themselves will allow them to ask for help when needed, aid them in setting personal boundaries, help them gain access to necessary resources, and more.
    - Teaching someone to say "Ma'am" or "Sir" when speaking to others may be polite, but it is not necessary or socially significant. Alternatively, teaching a shy person public speaking skills is socially significant.

  - **See:** Behavior

- **Spontaneous Recovery**

  - **Translation:**

    - When a behavior someone used to engage in that was not rewarded anymore has started happening again

  - **Examples:**

    - You have been ignoring your ex's attempts to contact you (e.g., texts and calls) for the past year. He hasn't tried to contact you in a while, but he starts texting you again.
    - An inmate at a prison almost successfully escaped. He has not tried to escape in a few months but attempted to jump the fence in the prison yard today.

  - **See:** Extinction and reinforcement

- **Stimulus**

  - **Translations:**

    - Anything you can sense and respond to
    - Something that causes a reaction or response in living organisms
    - Something around us that makes us feel or act a certain way

- **Examples:**

  - The waves crashing on the beach outside of Rose's hotel room help her relax.
  - Gary smells his mother's pasta sauce and it makes him excited about dinner.

- **See:** Discriminative stimulus, stimulus control, stimulus fading, and stimulus generalization

- **Stimulus Control**

  - **Translation:**

    - When a signal tells you to behave a certain way
    - When something in the environment reliably influences behavior

  - **Examples:**

    - At the beginning of a race, runners will start to run as soon as they hear the shot of the gun. The gunshot has stimulus control over them starting to run.
    - When someone wears a ring on their left ring finger, Jake knows this usually means this person is engaged or married to their partner. This deters Jake from asking this person on a date.

  - **See:** Behavior, discriminative stimulus, stimulus, and stimulus fading

- **Stimulus Fading**

  - **Translation:**

    - Slowly changing the things we can sense (e.g., how much we are exposed to or how quickly they are presented to us) that control our behavior to increase the likelihood of a desired response happening.

  - **Examples:**

    - Franco refuses to eat green foods. His mom slowly adds small amounts of green food to his meals. Over time, Franco is able to eat an entire helping of garlic broccoli at dinner. You go, Franco!
    - We have glow lights in our bedroom, which we turn on at night. They slowly dim every few minutes, ultimately turning completely off leaving the room dark. This helps us get ready to go to sleep. In the morning, they slowly get brighter to help us wake up.

  - **See:** Stimulus, stimulus control, and stimulus generalization

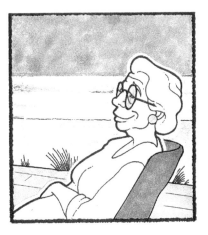

Figure 10.3 "You can hear, see, feel, smell, and even taste the waves at the beach, making them stimuli in your environment."

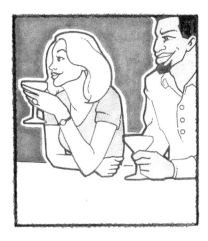

Figure 10.4 "Stimulus control can explain when you know when and when not to approach a possible mate. These are reliable signals in your environment that tell you how to respond."

- **Stimulus Generalization**

  - **Translation:**

    - Responding to different things in the environment in the same way

  - **Examples:**

    - After being burned on the stove, you keep your hands away from anything with a flame (i.e., a bonfire, a candle, and the stove being turned on).
    - After Anne was taught to write with a pencil, she was seen writing with pens, markers, chalk, or even crayons.

  - **See:** Generalization, response generalization, stimulus, and stimulus fading

- **Systematic Desensitization**

  - **Translation:**

    - Slowly exposing someone to triggering things and teaching them calming strategies so they become less anxious or fearful of them in the future

  - **Examples:**

    - Police departments use systematic desensitization training to help their new officers become tolerant of being struck by another person or having to strike another in a physical confrontation (Klugiewicz, 2010).
    - Zach is extremely fearful of public speaking. He has to present in front of one of his college classes coming up. Zach's therapist has created a plan to slowly build up his tolerance to speaking in front of larger groups of people, as well as teaching him calming strategies to use while he presents.

  - **See:** Habituation and stimulus fading

References

Bailey, J. S. (1991). Marketing behavior analysis requires different talk. *Journal of Applied Behavior Analysis, 24*(3), 445–448. https://doi.org/10.1901/jaba.1991.24-445

Branch, M. N., & Vollmer, T. R. (2004). Two suggestions for the verbal behavior(s) of organisms (i.e., authors). *The Behavior Analyst, 27*(1), 95–98. https://doi.org/10.1007/BF03392094

Critchfield, T. S. (2014). Ten rules for discussing behavior analysis. *Behavior Analysis in Practice, 7*(2), 141–142. https://doi.org/10.1007/s40617-014-0026-z

Friman, P. C. (2004). Up with this I shall not put: 10 reasons why I disagree with Branch and Vollmer on behavior used as a count noun. *The Behavior Analyst, 27*(1), 99–106. https://doi.org/10.1007/BF03392095

Foxx R. M. (1996). Translating the covenant: The behavior analyst as ambassador and translator. *The Behavior analyst, 19*(2), 147–161. https://doi.org/10.1007/BF03393162

Hayes, S. C. (1991). The limits of technological talk. *Journal of Applied Behavior Analysis, 24*(3), 417–420. https://doi.org/10.1901/jaba.1991.24-417

Hineline, P. N. (1980). The language of behavior analysis: Its community, its functions, and its limitations. *Behaviorism, 8*(1), 67–86.

Klugiewicz, G. T. (2010). *Desensitization training helps officers stay in the fight: people aren't born with the ability to hit and be hit – they have a sensory inhibition that every officer must learn to overcome.* Police1. https://www.police1.com/close-quarters-combat/articles/desensitization-training-helps-officers-stay-in-the-fight-JZVaTrpBFszjNzVc/

Lindsley, O. R. (1991). From technical jargon to plain English for application. *Journal of Applied Behavior Analysis, 24*(3), 449–458. https://doi.org/10.1901/jaba.1991.24-449

Marshall, K. B. (2021). *The impact of behavior analysis jargon on the effective training of stakeholders* [Doctoral dissertation, Endicott College]. ProQuest. https://www.proquest.com/docview/2571066257?pq-origsite=gscholar&fromopenview=true

Risley, T. R. (1975). Certify procedures not people. In W. Scott Wood (ed.), *Issues in evaluating behavior modification* (pp. 159–181). Research Press.

Schlinger, H. D., Blakely, E., Fillhard, J., & Poling, A. (1991). Defining terms in behavior analysis: Reinforcer and discriminative stimulus. *The Analysis of Verbal Behavior*, *9*, 153–161. https://doi.org/10.1007/BF03392869

11 Others Selling Behavior Science

Many different professionals have written books and produced content about behavior science over the years. Chris Voss, former lead international kidnapping negotiator for the Federal Bureau of Investigation (FBI) (The Black Swan Group, n.d.), and Tahl Raz, a New York Times best-selling writer and award-winning journalist (Raz, n.d.), wrote *Never Split the Difference*, a book that teaches readers how to master negotiating strategies. James Clear, who wrote the book *Atomic Habits*, instructs his readers how to make small changes to their habits that yield big results. *Nudge: Improving Decisions About Health, Wealth, and Happiness* by Richard H. Thaler, one of the founders of behavioral economics (UChicago News, n.d.), and Cass R. Sunstein, former White House Office Administrator for Information and Regulatory Affairs and the founder and director of the behavioral economics and public policy program at Harvard Law School (Harvard Kennedy School, n.d.), use behavior economics to coach people how to make better daily decisions to improve their lives. There are also many social media influencers who speak solely about how to create healthy habits and break bad ones. Shelby Sacco (@shelbysacco5) on TikTok shows her 1.5 million followers how to use cues and rewards to start new habits.

All of these individuals have one common denominator: they all speak basically so everyone can understand their message about behavior science. Rarely do they use jargon, if ever. For instance, For instance, James Clear has changed terms such as "motivating operations," to "cravings" and "behavior chaining" to "habit stacking." (Clear, 2018). Additionally, all of these books and platforms have been incredibly profitable. The books *Atomic Habits* and *Nudge: Improving Decisions About Health, Wealth, and Happiness* have both been labeled New York Times bestsellers. *Never Split the Difference* has been labeled a Wall Street Journal bestseller. They all make the language accessible and easy for their consumers to understand. Behavior analysts should be the best people to speak on the topic of behavior science, but without using the proper terminology, the information falls on deaf ears. Imagine the impact we can have once we start to talk like James Clear or Shelby Sacco. The possibilities are endless.

Terms and Translations

- **Tact**
  - **Translation:**
    - Labeling things

DOI: 10.4324/9781003439776-11

- **Examples:**

  - If I were to see Harry Styles walking down the street with my friends, I would probably scream, "That's Harry Styles!"
  - Stanley sees flames coming from the break room toaster and yells, "Fire!"

- **See:** Verbal behavior

- **Target Behavior**

  - **Translations:**

    - The behavior/habit/response of interest
    - The behavior/habit/response you are attempting to change
    - The skill you are attempting to teach or coach someone

  - **Examples:**

    - Carson teaches her clients to give compliments about someone's makeup instead of saying, "What's on your face?"
    - Hans teaches his granddaughter to put cardboard items in the recycling bin instead of the garbage.

  - **See:** Behavior

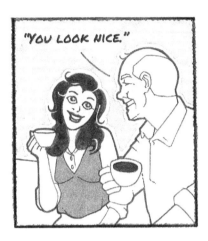

Figure 11.1 "A behavior analyst can teach their clients any significant skill, such as how to give simple compliments to others."

- **Task Analysis**

  - **Translations:**

    - A list of directions on how to perform a specific skill or routine
    - Breaking down a skill or routine into small steps to complete it

  - **Examples:**

    - Billy teaches his client how to make eggplant parmesan. He breaks the recipe down into small steps to make the process easier for his client to complete. Billy starts with the first step, which is washing the eggplant. Then, he teaches his client the rest of the steps.
    - The list of directions Google Maps gives you to reach your destination.

  - **See:** Chaining, behavior chain with limited hold, backward chaining, backward chaining with leaps ahead, forward chaining, and total task chaining

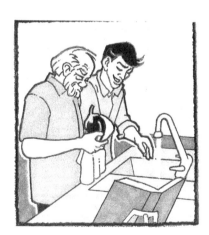

Figure 11.2 "A behavior analyst teaching his client how to make a new recipe."

- **Token Economy**

  - **Translation:**

    - A system for earing points, tokens, or other rewards to later exchange for larger rewards

  - **Examples:**

    - If Jake marks on his calendar at least three days that he worked out in a single week, he can reward himself with a margarita at the end of the third day.
    - In the book *Harry Potter*, each house earns points, which go toward winning the house cup at the end of the year.

  - **See:** Backup reinforcers and reinforcement

- **Topography**

  - **Translations:**

    - How a behavior looks
    - The visual appearance of an action

  - **Examples:**

    - Carson is working with athletes to better their running form. The topography is how the athletes move their arms and legs when they run.
    - The form of a child's tantrum can look like them screaming, crying, and dropping to the floor. An adult's tantrum can look like them writing an email that starts off with, "Per your last email," or yelling at a customer service representative and saying, "I demand to speak to your manager!"

  - **See:** Behavior

- **Total Task Chaining**

  - **Translation:**

    - Receiving instructions for each step of a routine from start to end during each teaching session

  - **Examples:**

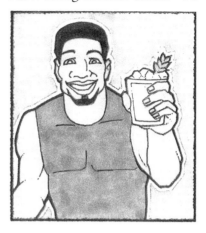

Figure 11.3 "Earning all of your checkmarks can be extremely motivating. Cheers!"

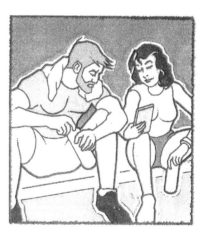

Figure 11.4 "The same action can look very different across people or over time for a single person, such as running. Running can look slow with moderate movement or fast with lots of arm and leg movement and heavy breathing."

- A new flight attendant needs help making the announcements to passengers boarding their flights. His trainer points to each line of the script while he starts the announcements and reminds him of any details he missed during every day of his training.
- In his spare time, Billy is a dance choreographer. When teaching his crew the steps to their dance routine, he shows them the entire routine and offers assistance for

the portions they need demonstrating every time they practice.

- **See:** Chaining, backward chaining, backward chaining with leaps ahead, behavior chain with limited hold, forward chaining, shaping, and task analysis

- **Transitive Conditioned Motivating Operation**

  - **Translation:**

    - When a part of the environment establishes another as a reward or punisher

  - **Examples:**

    - Bobby needing a ticket to get into the Beatles cover band concert
    - Rose needing scissors to open a package with her new shoes in it

  - **See:** Abolishing operation, conditioned motivating operation, establishing operation, motivating operation, reflexive conditioned motivating operation, unconditioned motivating operation

- **Treatment Integrity/Procedural Fidelity**

  - **Translation:**

    - Testing how accurate someone is at administering or implementing strategies or a plan

  - **Examples:**

    - A behavior analyst tests to see if a manager is giving out the employee of the month award every month or not
    - Observing to see if a coach is correcting their players after they make a mistake or not

  - **See:** Interobserver agreement (IOA) and treatment

- **Unconditioned**

  - **Translations:**

    - Not learned
    - Being born with this instinct

  - **Examples:**

    - Squinting when you look into the sun

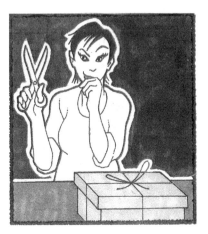

Figure 11.5 "One is not born knowing you might need scissors to open a box. You have learned this over time, which means this is a conditioned motivator."

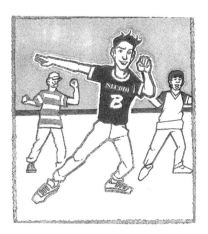

Figure 11.6 "When a choreographer gives his dancers directions on each step of their new routine every time they practice, he would be using total task chaining."

- Sneezing when dust gets in your nose
- **See:** Unconditioned motivating operation and unconditioned stimulus
- **Unconditioned Motivating Operation**
  - **Translations:**
    - Unlearned craving
    - Unlearned motivation
    - Unlearned motivator
    - Something you were born motivated by, which can alter how powerful rewards/punishers are and how often behaviors occur
  - **Examples:**

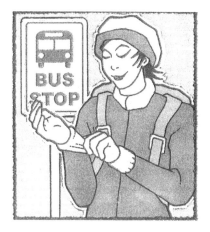

    - Michael Scarn has not been intimate with another person in a few years. During this period of time, his motivation to watch the show, *Bridgerton,* and read the book series, *Fifty Shades of Grey,* which have a lot of sexual content, has increased significantly during this time.
    - Waiting outside for the bus when it's snowing may motivate Rose to put gloves on. Due to the cold temperatures, this can make having gloves very rewarding.
  - **See:** Abolishing operation, conditioned motivating operation, establishing operation, and motivating operation

Figure 11.7 "Being cold can motivate you to search for a heated area, buy a new parka, or put on gloves to keep your hands warm."

- **Unconditioned Stimulus**
  - **Translation:**
    - Anything you can sense that makes behavior happen without prior learning history.
  - **Examples:**
    - Eating sour foods or drinks can make someone pucker.
    - Hot weather can make someone sweat.
  - **See:** Unconditioned and stimulus

For Further Reading

Clear, J. (2018) *Atomic habits: An easy and proven way to build good habits and break bad ones.* Avery, an imprint of Penguin Random House.

Rowling, J. K. (1999). *Harry Potter and The Sorcerer's Stone.* Scholastic.

Kee, C. (2022). *After years of disordered eating, walking and 1 healthy eating hack turned her life around: Shelby Sacco went viral on TikTok for sharing how she lost 25 pounds by eating healthy 60-80% of the week. She struggled for years with disordered eating.* Today. https://www.today.com/health/diet-fitness/walking-1-healthy-eating-hack-helped-lose-25-pounds-rcna37629

Thaler, R. H., & Sunstein, C. R. (2008). *Nudge: Improving decisions about health, wealth, and happiness*. Yale University Press.
Voss, C., & Raz, T. (2017). *Never split the difference*. Random House Business Books.

References

Harvard Kennedy School. (n.d). *Cass Sunstein*. Harvard Kennedy School. https://www.hks.harvard.edu/faculty/cass-sunstein
Raz, T. (n.d). *About Tahl Raz*. LinkedIn. https://www.linkedin.com/in/tahlraz.
The Black Swan Group. (n.d.). *About Chris Voss*. The Black Swan Group. https://www.blackswanltd.com/chris-voss
UChicago News. (n.d.). *Richard Thaler*. *https://news.uchicago.edu/profile/richard-thaler#:~:text=Considered%20to%20be%20one%20of,Prof.*

12 Life Changing Tips

Over the years of being a behavior analyst, I've learned so much about why people and animals do what they do and how to be successful in this career. Here are some of the most life-changing tips to help readers understand others and yourself better, whether you work in behavior science or not:

- **Be the best listener and observer in the room.**
  - If you're too busy talking or getting caught up in your own head, you'll miss extremely important details about what is happening right in front of your face. Give your mouth a break and let your eyes and ears do the work.

- **Observe before making moves.**
  - One of the biggest mistakes I've made as a behavior analyst is worrying about failing before I even started the job. I noticed I did this when I worked with my first clients and still do it to this day. I would see a behavior that needed correction (e.g., someone using the wrong phrase, employees gossiping and a pitcher releasing the ball incorrectly), then I would start to internally have a panic attack because I would be fearful about potentially not knowing how to fix the problem. What helps me break this cycle is taking a deep breath, or four, then watching the behavior happen again with a purely observational mindset and documenting what I see. This is especially important when you are seeing a behavior for the first time. You can't change something you don't know anything about. Observe, observe again, and again, document, review your findings, and then draw conclusions. If after you've gone through all of these steps and are still unsure about how to move forward, ask for help! Some people can't wait to be of aid to another. It's an incentive to them. These techniques help me pinpoint the issues with a calm headspace and avoid getting all worked up trying to create a plan on how I'm going to change the problem before I truly know from where the issue is coming.

- **Look at people's eyes when trying to understand their motives.**
  - You can see where a person's focus goes, how their eyebrows move, or if their attention is somewhere else. This is another detail that can be easily missed if you're busy kibitzing or overthinking your own actions.

- **Consistency is the first key.**
  - Whether you are starting a new habit, getting rid of a bad habit, or maintaining a current skill, consistency is your best friend. For example, if your expectation is to

DOI: 10.4324/9781003439776-12

take the garbage out every Tuesday night or text your sister at least once per day, like me, consistency is a requirement to keep the habit going. No one has ever mastered anything by just doing it once in a while.

- **There's always a reason.**

  - Every behavior has a reason for happening. There is always something maintaining it. Nothing ever happens *out of the blue.*

- **Patience is the second key.**

  - Have patience when changing behavior. Even if some errors happen, which they will, trust the process and your plan because it is just that, a process. Behavior change is not as easy as taking a magic potion and immediately seeing the results you want. Goals do not get mastered overnight. "Behavior changes gradually" (Critchfield, 2014, p. 141).

- **Treat yourself**

  - Treating yourself for meeting goals is a helpful and evidence-based strategy, also known as reinforcement, so do it! Do it consistently, and tell other people about your goals. They can assist in holding you accountable.

- **One goal**

  - Change one behavior or set one goal at a time. This will be much easier for you, and there will be less details to keep track of over time.

- **Short-term versus long-term goals**

  - Bookmark this page for your next New Year's resolution. When setting goals, make sure you have long-term AND SHORT-TERM GOALS. Your long-term goal is your ultimate, final destination for what you want (e.g., being fluent in Spanish, working out five days per week, eating a vegan diet). Your short-term goals are the small ones that keep you on track and motivated to keep going (e.g., learning one new Spanish word per day and doing one 30-minute workout per week). The best way I've found to choose your short-term goals is to work backwards from your long-term goal. For instance, I have a long-term goal of being able to play the ukulele without needing sheet music for any song. Currently, I don't know anything about the ukulele. I just know I love the way it sounds and want to play it well. My short-term goals could look like the following: playing one cord on the ukulele, playing four cords, being able to play one song, being able to play three songs, etc. If you only have a long-term goal, which is where most of us start, it's easy to become discouraged and lose motivation. The mastery of your little stepping stone goals is where the magic happens.

- **Effective communication is one of the best ways to avoid issues.**

  - This can help with the simplest problems, like your friend forgetting what time your brunch reservation is, to more complicated ones, such as negotiating with terrorists to release hostages. Effective communication with lasting results was the exact reason for creating this book. It works and brings people together.

Terms and Translations

- **Variable Interval Schedule of Reinforcement**

  - **Translation:**

    - Fluctuating amounts of time before a behavior/response is rewarded

  - **Examples:**

    - During a golf team's practice, a coach will have his players to take breaks about every 20 minutes. The next week, the breaks will come about every 30 minutes of practicing.
    - PJ is at a casino in Las Vegas playing a slot machine. About every 10–15 minutes, a waiter comes over to PJ to ask her if she'd like a drink refill.

  - **See:** Reinforcement and schedules of reinforcement

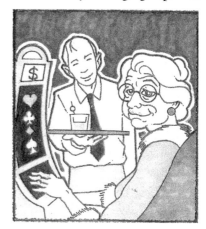

Figure 12.1 "Casinos are so accommodating to their customers who spend more time at the slot machines."

- **Variable Ratio Schedule of Reinforcement**

  - **Translation:**

    - A fluctuating number of behaviors/responses before a reward is delivered

  - **Examples:**

    - Jake receives an extra 100 points from his favorite cannabis dispensary about every three times he buys products there.
    - When scrolling on social media, the platform shows you content from one of your favorite categories about every seven videos you watch.

  - **See:** Reinforcement and schedule of reinforcement

- **Verbal Behavior**

  - **Translation:**

    - Communication behavior

  - **Examples:**

    - A husband signs to his partner saying, "I love you."
    - A baby points to her bottle to signal to her father that she wants a drink.

  - **See:** Mand, tact, intraverbal, echoic, and functional communication training

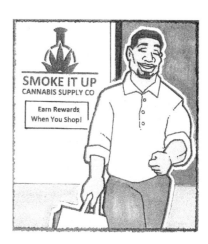

Figure 12.2 "When you are rewarded fairly often for shopping at your favorite stores, you will probably go there more frequently."

- **Whole Interval Recording**
  - **Translation:**
    - Only recording that a behavior happened if it occurred during an entire block of time
  - **Examples:**
    - A teacher wants to increase her class' on-task behavior during independent reading time. She sets her timer for five minutes. If the whole class reads for the entire five minutes, she records the reading behavior happened. If any class members need reminders to keep doing their work, she does not record the behavior occurring.
    - Morgan, a doctoral level behavior analyst, has been hired by a court to increase jurors' behavior of attending to the presentation of case information. If the entire jury keeps their eyes on the people speaking or are taking notes during a specific time period, Morgan will record that the attending behavior happened.
  - **See:** Data, direct measurement, and discontinuous measurement

For Further Reading

Clear, J. (2018) *Atomic habits: An easy & proven way to build good habits and break bad ones.* Avery, an imprint of Penguin Random House.

Cooper, J. O., Heron, T. E., & Heward, W. L. (eds.). (2007). *Applied behavior analysis* (2nd ed.). Merrill Prentice Hall.

Center for Disease Control. (2018, August). Data collection methods for program evaluation: Observation. Retrieved from https://www.cdc.gov/healthyyouth/evaluation/pdf/brief16.pdf

Ghaemmaghami, M., Hanley, G. P., & Jessel, J. (2021). Functional communication training: From efficacy to effectiveness. *Journal of Applied Behavior Analysis, 54*(4), 122–143. https://doi.org/10.1002/jaba.762

Fryling, M. J., Wallace, M. D., & Yassine, J. N. (2012). Impact of treatment integrity on intervention effectiveness. *Journal of Applied Behavior Analysis, 45*(2), 449–453. https://doi.org/10.1901/jaba.2012.45-449

Hayes, S. C., Rosenfarb, I., Wulfert, E., Munt, E. D., Korn, Z., & Zettle, R. D. (1985). Self-reinforcement effects: An artifact of social standard setting?. *Journal of Applied Behavior Analysis, 18*(3), 201–214. https://doi.org/10.1901/jaba.1985.18-201

Iwata, B. A., Dorsey, M. F., Slifer, K. J., Bauman, K. E., & Richman, G. S. (1994). Toward a functional analysis of self-injury. *Journal of Applied Behavior Analysis, 27*(2), 197–209. https://doi.org/10.1901/jaba.1994.27-197

Epstein, R. (1997). Skinner as self-manager. *Journal of Applied Behavior Analysis, 30*(3), 545–568. https://doi.org/10.1901/jaba.1997.30-545

Seymour, M. A. (2002). Case study: A retired athlete runs down comeback road. In R. W. Malott & H. Harrison (eds.), *I'll stop procrastinating when I get around to it: Plus other cool ways to succeed in school and life using behavior analysis to get your act together* (p. 7–12). MI. Department of Psychology. Western Michigan University.

Voss, C., & Raz, T. (2017). *Never split the difference.* Random House Business Books.

Reference

Critchfield, T. S. (2014). Ten rules for discussing behavior analysis. *Behavior Analysis in Practice, 7*(2), 141–142. https://doi.org/10.1007/s40617-014-0026-z

Index

For Product Safety Concerns and Information please contact our EU
representative GPSR@taylorandfrancis.com
Taylor & Francis Verlag GmbH, Kaufingerstraße 24, 80331 München, Germany